STRONG HEART, SHARP MIND

STRONG HEART, SHARP MIND

6-STEP PROGRAM THAT REVERSES HEART DISEASE AND HELPS PREVENT ALZHEIMER'S

JOSEPH C. PISCATELLA AND
DR. MARWAN SABBAGH, MD

WITH JOHN HANC

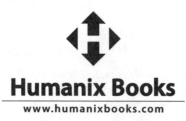

Humanix Books

www.humanixbooks.com

Humanix Books

STRONG HEART, SHARP MIND
Copyright © 2022 by Joseph C. Piscatella and Marwan Sabbagh, MD
All rights reserved

Humanix Books, P.O. Box 20989, West Palm Beach, FL 33416, USA
www.humanixbooks.com | info@humanixbooks.com

Humanix Books is a division of Humanix Publishing, LLC. Its trademark, consisting of the words "Humanix Books," is registered in the Patent and Trademark Office and in other countries.

Disclaimer: The information presented in this book is not specific medical advice for any individual and should not substitute medical advice from a health professional. If you have (or think you may have) a medical problem, speak to your doctor or a health professional immediately about your risk and possible treatments. Do not engage in any care or treatment without consulting a medical professional.

ISBN: 9-781-63006-193-7 (Hardcover)
ISBN: 9-781-63006-194-4 (E-book)

Printed in the United States of America
10   9   8   7   6   5   4   3   2   1

*To my wife, Bernie, my most constructive
critic, ardent supporter, and best friend.*

The journey with her has been a gift from God.

—J. C. P.

*To the love of my life, Ida, whose
patience, love, and undying support
carry me and inspire me.*

—M. S.

Contents

Foreword

WE ALL LIVE IN a world of wires and medical treatments. Huh, you say? What's the connection between wires and treatments? Well, hear me out.

Wires connect our computers' central processing units to our monitors. In braces, wires help shift the position of teeth. On skyscrapers, they keep window washers from falling. In bras, they do the same for breasts. Even in a society with cell phones and wireless internet access, we still rely on wires for so many things. Strip a house or new building of its siding, drywall, and insulation, and you'll see a labyrinth-like system of wires that snakes through the framing to supply power and internet connections to every room. Everything flows in and out of a central station—your fuse box—but ends with you connecting something, whether it be a light, a TV, or a cell phone charger. Without a strong power source, your house would merely be a three-bedroom, two-and-a-half-bath turtle shell. Your anatomical fuse box—your brain—has the same kind of responsibility. But your brain and its parts, in the Rodney Dangerfield sense, "get no respect"—until they need treatment.

In fact, hearts—the other power source—get all the attention. No one sings, "I left my brain in San Francisco." No one exchanges brains on Valentine's Day. And when was the last time you ever played blackjack with a queen of cerebellums?

As for treatments, that's how we in medicine are trained—that is, how to retrain a patient's left arm to function after a stroke, how to take away the keys after you've lost the ability to drive safely, or how to treat a heart attack or chest pain. In medical school and residencies, we doctors have largely been trained to identify and treat disease. It is the same for your brain and your heart—we in America (and all the developed world) see our doctors about our heart or our brain when something has happened to their function.

Ironically, we medical providers are compensated much better for treating disease than for preventing it—it is more lucrative to put a stent in a blood vessel in a heart or in a blood vessel to the brain than to teach you how to prevent that heart attack or stroke to begin with.

Now, you'd think that as someone who ran a large set of operating rooms and intensive care units, that's how I'd think—that is, about treatments. But the most important thing about avoiding days in the ICU postsurgery is staying physiologically young, having a RealAge many years younger than your calendar age. And the key organs to take care of—to prevent disease or even reverse it—are your brain and nervous system and your heart and cardiovascular system. The amazing thing Joe Piscatella and Dr. Marwan Sabbagh show in this book is that the same six key "wellness" strategies for keeping your brain healthy also prevent heart disease. (No, they didn't talk about alcohol, but few things that are good for one organ aren't good for preventing disease and the need for treatment of the other organ.)

For twenty years, I have held a conference eponymous with my name focused on wellness, healthy aging, and longevity. Concurrent with these conferences, wellness, healthy aging, and longevity have been growing exponentially. It makes sense, from a policy and public health standpoint (and for you as an individual), to *prevent* disease rather than treat it. That's precisely what these conferences teach health professionals and the laypeople who participate.

And while I have been such a strong proponent of making your RealAge younger with healthy choices (so much so that I wrote several bestselling books—*RealAge* and *You: The Owner's Manual*—and have served at the Cleveland Clinic as its first chief wellness officer), I am envious of the great way Joe and Marwan put this book and the brain-and-heart prevention plan together. Publications from Medicare database studies, the Nurses' Health Study, the Health Professionals Follow-Up Study, and the Alameda County and Whitehall and Swedish Men's studies (and I could go on for a full page) indicate that 75 percent of all diseases after age eighteen are preventable through simple lifestyle choices. And maybe more than 50 percent of dementia and 80 percent of arterial heart disease—those are diseases of the wires—need no treatments if you make those simple lifestyle choices Joe and Dr. Sabbagh detail in this book.

Heart attacks—despite all the efforts and despite the sizeable reduction of mortality from treatment in the past three decades—are still the leading cause of death. And dementia is epidemic and increasing. But beyond the prevention of heart disease, we have begun to crack the secrets of the brain and preventing brain disease. The brain was largely held as sacred and untouchable until recently. The degenerative diseases of the brain were considered to be unidirectional and terminal. But Dr. Sabbagh and his colleagues discovered that the brain is much more dynamic and its diseases much more preventable than previously thought. There is much more in common among the wires of the heart and brain—when you prevent dementia, you prevent heart disease, whether by social connections and passions (and other stress-reduction programs), physical activity, food choices that taste great, toxin avoidance, or good sleep habits.

Joe Piscatella and Marwan Sabbagh, MD, link wires and treatments in this book. They detail in *Strong Heart, Sharp Mind* that the same thing that keeps the wires functioning reduces the need for treatment: prevention. And probably surprisingly, they show that what's good for keeping your heart pumping also keeps your memories and passions alive. They give you a really great plan to follow. This book can help many and hopefully will help you and yours for years to come. Buy a copy for each and all in your family; I'm going to encourage my patients to do so. It is that important and that great a plan.

Michael Roizen, MD
Professor, Cleveland Clinic Lerner College of Medicine at Case Western Reserve University and Chief Wellness Officer Emeritus, Cleveland Clinic

Introduction

ON HIS 1989 ALBUM *Full Moon Fever,* Tom Petty sang about "a mind, with a heart of its own."

Regardless of precisely what the late rocker meant in the lyrics of that cryptic song, he was musing about a relationship that many have speculated upon over the centuries. Hearts and minds are often linked—as in that very phrase itself, the title of a 1974 Academy Award–winning documentary about the Vietnam War, where the phrase "winning hearts and minds" became synonymous with failed American efforts to garner the emotional and intellectual support of the populace behind the conflict.

Philosophers and physicians have long debated the primacy between the heart and brain or, more broadly, between emotions and reason. Aristotle famously declared the heart as the seat of consciousness, making the brain essentially, well . . . an afterthought. Others felt the same way, as what has been termed a *cardio-centric* view prevailed for centuries: "The heart has its reasons, which reason does not know," Pascal wrote in 1675—about fifty years after William Harvey figured out that the heart was not a sentient organism but essentially a marvelously designed pump. Harvey's discovery, wrote the University of Calgary's Dr. Steven W. A. Reynolds, "helped end the notion that the heart was intelligent and directed the functions of other organs."

Or did it? Harvey himself continued to refer to the heart as the "king" or "sun" of the body. He also maintained that, in addition to being a wonderful mechanism for circulating blood, the heart was the seat of emotions and did not challenge its metaphysical role. "To this day," Reynolds writes, "the heart remains a symbol of the soul and of emotion and the stylized heart symbol evokes images of love and passion."

That's the way it has continued ever since: the two vital organs, viewed as shorthand for the extremes of human behavior; opposite sides of the spectrum—emotion versus reason; passion versus logic; impulsive action versus deliberate, planned decisions. Even in the scientific community, the heart and the brain have long been viewed as separate. Equally important to the functioning of a human being, yes, but studied and treated by specialists working in their own branches of medicine, with their own journals and research papers, and without much thought to the interconnection of the two most vital organs.

It's important to note that much has changed in our understanding of both the brain and the heart in the past few decades. In the next chapter, we will discuss how our perceptions and understanding of both—in their separate disciplines of cardiology and neurology—have evolved.

But as significant as these new insights are, what's exciting to us is how in the last ten years, researchers have begun to take a fresh look at the heart-brain nexus. The Heart and Brain Conference, held in Paris in 2012, brought an interdisciplinary approach to the important question of how heart and brain health were related, along with the inverse—that is, how dysfunction in one could be linked to problems in the other. At that first forward-looking conference, cardiologists and neurologists discussed the common diseases that each treated separately—in particular stroke. Since then, there has been a recognition of even greater overlap in the two areas.

"An intimate and underestimated relationship" is how University of Amsterdam pathologist Mat Daemen so artfully put it in an influential 2013 paper. He predicted that as our society ages, the link between a dysfunctional heart and a cognitively impaired brain could become a vital healthcare priority in the future. With an estimated 108.7 million Americans now fifty and older, the significance of this link becomes critical—particularly as we contemplate the rising numbers in two diseases that, despite the recent

COVID-19 pandemic, are the ones most would agree still pose the greatest long-term public health challenges to an aging America: heart disease, the nation's number-one killer, and Alzheimer's disease, the most feared affliction and one that itself is reaching epidemic proportions.

According to a recent survey of Baby Boomers, 95 percent felt themselves either unprepared for a diagnosis of Alzheimer's or that they would find life "not worth living" with it.

But mounting evidence suggests a much closer relationship between these two diseases than previously thought. Even more compelling is the research showing that something can be done about it, that steps can be taken—some familiar, others new—to maximize and improve heart *and* brain health together.

"It is time for a more integrative view to the heart brain connection," declared Dr. Daemen in 2013. "We believe that time is now, as heart disease continues to take its toll . . . as Alzheimer's continues its steady climb . . . as readers 50 and over, perhaps reminded of the importance of adopting better health habits during the current epidemic, are looking to take steps to ensure their well-being and quality of life for decades to come."

Hence the urgent need for a book that can explain this new interconnection of a healthy heart and brain, one that can show you how to forge the vital link.

This is that book.

STRONG HEART, SHARP MIND

Strong Heart, Sharp Mind relies on the latest science to tie together heart and brain health. But in addition to providing information, we offer a proven program to optimize that critical junction—one that is based on the latest research as well as the experience of two professionals who have dedicated their lives and careers to helping people recognize and adopt the behaviors needed to protect them from heart and Alzheimer's disease.

Our book will combine science and how-to; information and inspiration, rendered through the first-person, motivational voice of Joe Piscatella; the authoritative scientific insights of Dr. Marwan Sabbagh; and prescriptive material developed by both along with award-winning book writer and journalist John Hanc—as well as insights from innovative and cutting-edge health, medical, and wellness practitioners around the world.

Together, we will blend science and solution in the form of a new, singular heart/brain-specific prescriptive program, developed for you by the authors and rooted in their work and experiences as well as that of other leading-edge thinkers and practitioners in this exciting new intersection of health and medicine.

WHAT'S THE CONNECTION?

Some say the reason behind the deep connection between the brain and heart is simple: blood flow.

It is true that both the heart and brain rely on large amounts of precisely controlled blood coursing through the veins and arteries to stay ticking and sparking at optimal levels. Many conditions affect the circulatory system including heart disease, stroke, diabetes and high blood pressures. Strokes, when they accumulate, can cause vascular dementia, one of the most common forms of dementia after Alzheimer's.

But physicians have understood the concept of blood circulation since the days of William Harvey. Now we are beginning to see other eye-opening connections between heart and brain—between the major diseases that affect both and the things that can be done to prevent, forestall, or ameliorate them. Consider the commonality of risk factors. In recent years, it has become apparent to those of us in the research community that the well-known risk factors for cardiovascular disease are very similar to those of Alzheimer's disease.

This wasn't true in the past. We didn't realize, for example, that both hypertension and type 2 diabetes, long known as culprits for cardiovascular disease, are also risk factors for Alzheimer's disease. We didn't understand that ApoE4 (the genetic signature associated with higher rates of Alzheimer's) is also implicated in heart disease.

We didn't know that elevated cholesterol—another well-known risk factor in heart disease—is linked to higher levels of amyloid, the substance that forms the brain tangles that are a hallmark of Alzheimer's.

These are profound discoveries—and exciting! Why exciting? Because think of just those three common risk factors for heart and brain health: hypertension, diabetes, elevated cholesterol. What do they have in common? They are all conditions that can be managed, controlled, and even, in some cases, reversed.

We'll show you why and how in the pages of this book.

CHAPTER 1

Our Evolving Understanding of the Heart and Brain

ACHIEVING WHAT WE CALL brain-body balance is not simply a question of saying "just do the same things you'd do for a healthy heart and you'll have a healthy brain."

Certainly, the building blocks are similar: exercise, diet, and so forth. But we are now learning that there are specific applications of these lifestyle applications—the right kind of exercise, the right combination of foods, the right approach to cognitive stimulation and activity—that can provide maximum benefit for the function of both of the vital organs, affording not only greater protection against cardiovascular disease and Alzheimer's disease but also improved health, vitality, and quality of life.

Outside of the research community, few have explored this connection. Think of it as a one-two punch of lifestyle interventions that can maximize heart-brain health.

The person with an optimal brain-body balance is also the one most likely to achieve an enormous *health span*. It's not only that your values look good on your blood-work (although that's important) or that you're someone who can now breathe easier over your lowered prospects of cardiovascular disease and Alzheimer's disease. The reader who follows the prescription in this book will quickly discover a new gear, a new level.

You will be at the top of your game—fully functioning, with a degree of mental sharpness and boundless energy allowing you to flourish in a fast-changing and challenging world, both at home and in your professional life.

That's the promise behind brain-body balance, behind optimizing the synergy between our two most vital organs: providing readers with a road map to achieve that new standard of health and longevity.

Before we get further into the convergence of heart and brain health, however, let's step back a moment and look at these vital organs *separately*. Specifically, let's look at how our understanding of both has changed in recent decades. In doing so, we will give you a better sense of who we are and how our own experiences in the worlds of heart and brain health have shaped our views.

Let's start with the heart, which of course is so central to our lives that it has become a synonym for the essence of an issue or problem—as in "the heart of the matter." Fittingly, it has been at the heart of Joe Piscatella's life and work—and few have a better perspective on the evolution of this essential organ and cardiovascular health than he does.

JOE'S JOURNEY: A DISHEARTENING DIAGNOSIS

"Go home, take two aspirin, and call me in the morning."

That was the advice my cardiologist gave me after an examination revealed that I had a blocked coronary artery.

It was 1977, and I was thirty-two years old and living in Lakewood, Washington, a suburb of Tacoma, with my wife, Bernie, and our two children, Anne, then six years old, and Joe, who was four. While my health was generally good, I was a few pounds overweight, I didn't really exercise regularly—few adults outside of professional athletes did in those days—and my diet was an all-American one for that era: I ate lots of red meat and processed foods and still drank milk ("For strong bones and healthy teeth!" we were told).

Also, although the term was just beginning to enter the parlance, I was under chronic stress caused by never seeming to have enough time between my family and my work.

That spring, Jimmy Carter was president, Abba's "Dancing Queen" was the number-one song on the charts, and in late May, a cheesy-sounding science fiction film was about to open (in only forty-three theaters nationwide) called *Star Wars*.

Every day for the first six months of 1977, I would get up, race out the door—generally without any breakfast to speak of—and head to my office. While my job with a regional business association was a good one, it was demanding. I was driving down to the state capital in Olympia daily and meeting with local legislators on behalf of our clients, mostly small and midsized Washington State businesses that—in the midst of the seventies recession and oil crisis—were struggling to stay afloat.

There was a lot of pressure on them and, thus, on me.

I'm sure I overlooked many telltale signs along the way that it was all taking a toll on my health. But I wasn't concerned in the least until, in June, I began to notice a shortness of breath and a low-grade but nagging chest pain that came while playing tennis. I complained to Bernie about it.

"Maybe you should go see the doctor" was her suggestion.

I responded to this sensible recommendation the way most guys would have: I dismissed it and chose to ignore the problem.

About a month later, on July 17, I was scheduled to play a singles match with my friend. It was a Friday. Doug was a colleague of mine at the business association, where we were fortunate enough to have flexible hours in the summer (nothing happened in the legislature on Fridays in July, anyway).

Doug was an amiable guy and a talented athlete. On the court, we were well-matched, as most of our games were close. While it was fun, we were also both competitive young men, so when I started feeling that fullness building in my chest again during the warm-up that day, I tried to work through it. This was male ego and testosterone at its best (or worst): real men didn't walk from competition because of a little tightness in the chest! Besides, there was a myriad of reasons to explain it away. My discomfort might have been the result of that cheeseburger I wolfed down for lunch the day before our match. Or maybe I was coming down with something. In the damp Northwest climate, it seemed like people were always getting colds.

Regardless, the game would go on. Besides, I rationalized, this feeling of fullness in my chest that I'd been experiencing in recent weeks usually abated. But this time the pressure continued and even got worse over the course of two hours.

Meanwhile, the sun broke through the clouds, and the temperatures soared. I was sweating, I felt queasy, and my chest was starting to hurt like hell. I probably didn't drink enough water (we didn't call it "hydrating" in the seventies). But of course, I couldn't show weakness, especially to another young Turk who worked in the same office. Somehow, I made it through the game. I might have even won a few sets.

When I got home and confessed to Bernie that I really wasn't feeling well but had played for two hours anyway, she put her foot down and told me to see our doctor. I went directly to his office, walked in without an appointment, and announced to his staff, "I have bronchitis. Can you look at my lungs?"

I was annoyed that my Friday plans had been thrown off, but I wasn't expecting more than a prescription for a couple pills or perhaps a gentle admonition to slow down a bit on the tennis court—after all, I was in my thirties now. Everybody knew that adults shouldn't push themselves too hard. That's how you got a heart attack, right?

For some reason, I was convinced that my problem was some kind of respiratory illness. That's what I told our doctor when I was ushered into the examination room. "Well, everything sounds fine there," he said after listening to my lungs with his stethoscope. "But as long as you're here, and since you had some chest pains, let's do an electrocardiogram."

I'm sure I rolled my eyes as if to say, "Really? Must we?" It seemed like a waste of time to me. After all, I had just had an EKG a few months earlier at my annual physical, and it showed no problems. But heck, this was the doctor, and you always did what the doctor said.

He strapped me up to what looked like a giant AM/FM radio with a teletype machine attached. As he watched my heart rhythms undulate across the page that came chattering out of the machine, I could see his expression change from nonchalance to concern.

"I want you to see a cardiologist, Joe," he said.

"OK," I said. "I'll make an appointment on Monday."

"No," he said gravely. "Now. Immediately. In fact, I'll drive you, because I don't want you behind the wheel of the car."

That got my attention. Especially the driving part. When did a doctor volunteer to drive a patient, even one he knew?

Answer: when the situation was dead serious.

The cardiologist, after a brusque examination, decided to do a cardiac catheterization—then a relatively new test. Today, the modern health-care system being what it is, you'd need to schedule such a test several weeks in advance. But things were different in 1977. He called the hospital across the street, and we strolled over together.

I was wheeled into the cardiac cath lab, then given mild anesthesia. The procedure involves inserting a flexible tube with a camera in the groin (now they can do it in the arm), which is then directed through the cardiovascular system so a cardiologist can check for plaque buildup. Contrast dye is used to make plaque blockages more visible.

I woke up in a recovery room a couple of hours later with a bandage around my groin. Bernie was there.

"How are you feeling?" she asked.

"What a day," I managed with a weak smile. "Tennis in the morning, anesthesia in the afternoon."

We were joined shortly by the cardiologist. Unlike my doctor, this specialist didn't mince words (as I would be reminded several times in my interactions with him).

He glanced down at some papers on a clipboard. Among them, I assumed, were the results of my exam.

"You have a significant blockage in your left coronary artery," he announced, and he paused. "Do you know what they call that?"

"Er . . . no," I said, as Bernie and I exchanged glances.

"The widow maker," he said. "In other words, you're a heart attack waiting to happen. I'm going to schedule you for bypass surgery in a couple of days."

Bernie's grip on my hand tightened, and I could see her eyes well up with tears. I took a deep breath (and it hurt—I guessed he was right).

Although it's today the most commonly performed cardiac surgery procedure (about two hundred thousand bypasses a year are performed in the United States, according to a 2018 study), this was still relatively new at the time. I knew next to nothing about coronary heart disease in general, much less a cutting-edge, cardiac surgical procedure. As we struggled to process what such an operation would involve and what this would mean for us going forward, I asked him, "Is there anything I should do in the meantime?"

That's when he told me to go home and take those two aspirins. Given the severity of my situation, the advice wasn't as absurd or dismissive as it may sound today. It was already recognized that aspirin was a clot buster. But still, it's a reminder of what has changed so profoundly in the diagnosis and treatment of heart disease—and what hasn't, as we'll discuss in upcoming chapters.

Some significant things have *not* changed. The essential anatomy of the heart has been mapped out and understood since the late seventeenth century. By the time I was being prepped for my bypass—a procedure first performed in 1960—we certainly knew a lot more about how to treat a condition like mine and how to repair damaged hearts than they did in the days of William Harvey. But when it came to prevention and management—when it came to the question of what happened after surgery in the 1970s—we might as well have still been in the 1600s.

Suffice it to say that one of the many striking differences in the way my situation was treated in 1977 versus how it would be in 2021 is that throughout that entire, unforgettable day and in the days and weeks that followed, I was not asked about what I ate or if I smoked. Nor was I questioned about my levels of physical activity or the kind of job I had. No one seemed at all interested in whether I'd had trouble sleeping or been anxious or whether I was under any undue stress or had suffered any kind of traumatic personal event.

I was fighting for my life, but no one seemed interested in the kind of life I was living.

What a difference four decades have made. If I had bypass surgery now, my physicians and other health professionals would want to know a lot more about me. And they would have enrolled me in a cardiac rehabilitation program, where diet, exercise, smoking and alcohol use, and mental outlook would all have been risk factors that would have been discussed and, if necessary, addressed. Because today we know how important all those factors are to heart disease—and heart health. While there have certainly been many remarkable advances in drug therapy, technology, and the techniques of cardiac surgery in the last half century, I think the most striking and sweeping change is in the emphasis today on the importance of prevention. Today we know that positive lifestyle habits can help you prevent, halt, and even reverse heart disease.

That's my cautionary tale from 1977. But the fact that I'm still here in 2021 to tell you the story is cause for optimism. That's what the last few decades have taught us. The fate of your heart and your health is not necessarily in your genes; it's in your hands.

And as Dr. Sabbagh will now explain, that may also be the case with our brains.

DR. SABBAGH: THE ACTIVE BRAIN

I come from a family of doctors. My father was a cardiac surgeon; my mom is a PhD; my uncle is a neurosurgeon. Doctors everywhere! It was just natural for me to want to follow in their footsteps. I recall as a child accompanying my dad on his rounds at the hospital near where we lived in Tucson, Arizona. When I was a teenager, he gave me a copy of *Gray's Anatomy*.

I also knew pretty early on exactly what kind of specialty I wanted to practice. Although we were fortunate enough to not have Alzheimer's in our family, I found myself fascinated by the disease. As a teenager, it seemed like the embodiment of everything scary about aging. I was also attracted to the fact that we seemed to know very little about how to treat it. My dad could fix hearts—and like many cardiac surgeons, he saved many lives. But Alzheimer's was different. There was no surgical procedure or even any medication that could reverse it. There seemed to be . . . nothing.

To a curious, aspiring physician, this seemed like a challenge. I began researching the disease at age eighteen as a premed student at the University of California, Berkeley. Later, on my first date with Ida Crocker, a young medical student, I told her that the study of this terrible disease was what I wanted to devote my life to.

Ida became Ida Crocker-Sabbagh, MD, a family medicine physician. We have two wonderful sons, and I have no regrets about my career focus. OK, well, maybe frustration that we haven't yet cured Alzheimer's, sure. But while that remains elusive, we *have* made enormous progress in our understanding of the disease and in our ability to manage it. We are now at the stage where, at least in some cases, we can look at Alzheimer's as more of a chronic condition as opposed to the debilitating "no prevention, no treatment, no cure" affliction that it was when I first got into the field.

As a budding neurologist in medical school, however, we didn't just study Alzheimer's. I had to learn about many diseases that affect the brain and neural system—Parkinson's, epilepsy, stroke, migraine headaches. And of course we learned a great deal about the brain itself and what researchers then knew about its structure, its operation, and its growth.

Much of this, as it turned out, was wrong.

In 1997, I became board certified in neurology and went to work studying and treating Alzheimer's patients at University of California, San Diego—where modern Alzheimer's research had really begun in the 1980s. I later went on to be director of clinical research and then director of the Banner Sun Health Research Institute in Arizona and spent three years at the Barrow Neurological Institute in Phoenix before going to Cleveland Clinic, where I am currently director of translational research at the Clinic's Lou Ruvo Center for Brain Health in Las Vegas.

When you become a subspecialist as I did, you have tunnel vision. It's almost impossible to stay current on every other aspect of your field. That's part of the reason neurologists, like most physicians, need to get recertified every ten years. While I understood the importance of these exams, when it was my time to get recertified in 2007 and 2017, I complained to anyone who would listen. "This is taking time away from my patients and my research," I grumbled. "Why do I need to take an exam at this point of my career?"

Ida, my friends, and my colleagues nodded politely.

As a researcher with nearly four hundred published articles, I'm deeply immersed in the changing science behind my specialty of Alzheimer's disease. But what I learned in preparation for my recertification exams was, pardon the pun, mind-blowing: the changes in neurology and brain science that have occurred since I was a medical student have been sweeping, almost breathtaking. I daresay there are few disciplines in medicine in which the corpus of knowledge, the underlying assumptions and principles, have changed so radically. With all due respect to my colleagues in cardiology and the wonderful advances they have made in preventing and treating coronary heart disease, as Joe just pointed out, our basic understanding of the heart's anatomy and how it pumps blood has not changed in many decades.

That's not the case with the human brain. The advent of new imaging techniques that allow us to observe and better understand how the brain works in action combined with our new insights into genetics have transformed our understanding of the brain and how it functions.

"A continuous stream of advances is shattering long-held notions about how the human brain works and what happens when it doesn't," wrote Dr. Nora Volkow in 2010. Those advances have continued unabated at the time of this writing, in part because of our decoding of the human genome—it's now estimated that at least a third of the twenty thousand different genes that make up the genome are primarily related to the brain. Along with our evermore advanced imaging techniques, which now allow us to actually watch the brain in action, new light continues to be shed on our understanding of this most complex of human organisms—starting with the way in which they evolve.

When I was in medical school, we learned that the brain develops rapidly in the first five years of life, then has another "growth spurt" in our teenage years. Young brains crackle with newly produced neurons and synapses, increasing efficiency and capacity. And then it comes to a screeching stop. The brain remains an immutable, "fixed" organ until advancing age causes an inevitable diminishment: all those brilliant, sparkling neurons, dissipating like embers on a dying fire.

At least, that was the dogma twenty-five to thirty years ago. As I've learned during my recertification—and seen in some of my patients—what I was taught then was wrong.

"For a long time, it has been assumed that brain plasticity peaks at [a] young age and then gradually decreases as one gets older," wrote the authors of a 2018 paper in the journal *Aging*. "This is also underscored by the expression that one cannot teach an old dog new tricks, implying that people who have become used to doing things in a particular way will not easily abandon their habits and change their behavior. Interestingly, thanks to tremendous advances in medical imaging techniques for assessment of brain structure and function, mounting evidence for lifelong brain plasticity has been generated over the past years."

Plasticity—meaning *moldable*. Meaning that the brain is now recognized as having an extraordinary ability to mold and modify its own structure and function.

Although there is some neural deterioration that occurs with age, we now understand that the brain has the capacity to increase activity and develop what neuroscientists call "neural scaffolding" to regulate cognitive function. This, notes the University of Texas's Denise Park, PhD, involves the development of alternate, complementary neural circuits by the brain, much as platforms—scaffolds—are erected to support and protect an older structure during building renovations.

So when you think about it, that phrase "Cathedrals of the Mind" might not be far off. Just like a Renaissance cathedral, whose magnificence can still be appreciated today after restoration, so too can the human brain be refurbished to near-original luster through its own recently discovered restorative process.

The development of these alternate systems is an example of the brain's plasticity. But what is the stimulus that prompts it to build that scaffolding—to restructure and rewire to create new and more efficient pathways?

Learning.

"Every time you learn something new, you create a new synapse," says the eminent Harvard neuroscientist and author Dr. Rudolph Tanzi, referring to the neural pathways that connect neurons. "The more synapses you make, the more you can lose . . . before you lose it!"

The implications of this give new credence, even urgency, to the concept of lifelong learning. Those who choose to put in the effort can learn to master new skills, accumulate new knowledge, and adapt new behaviors, regardless of how old they are—and in doing so, they will be building up a neural reserve that can offset or delay the effects of aging.

That's an enormous change in our understanding of what's possible—not only in the deepest recesses of our brain but in our day-to-day lives.

One last dive into the new world of brain science: specifically, into the emergence of entire new subdisciplines that have sprung up in response to the avalanche of new data and that are now helping us study not only the brain but other organs and organisms. One group of these new fields are known as the "omics"—subsets of genomics, the new biological science that deals with the discovery and noting of all the sequences in the entire genome of a particular organism (and in our case, the particularly complex one known as the human brain).

Among the omics is a subdiscipline known as proteomics. This studies the structure and function of proteins that are responsible for many tasks at the cellular and genetic levels. Another is transcriptomics, which looks at ribonucleic acid—RNA—the messenger that carries instructions from the DNA. Yet another is epigenetics, which is the study of how the genome responds to environmental changes such as diet, sleep, and stress.

And then there's metabolomics (labeled "the final frontier" in a 2012 article in *Genomic Medicine*), which study metabolomes—compounds that affect the traits and characteristics of an organism.

Luckily, my board recertification doesn't require me to say "metabolomes" three times fast. But you get the point: it's a whole new world for those of us who study the brain or, as I do, one aspect or disease affecting it.

As I tell my patients, what these advances in brain science mean is that we should not take the so-called inevitable diseases commonly associated with aging as a fait accompli. I also push back at the idea that getting old must necessarily involve frailty, a dimming of cognitive skills, an inability to perform basic functions. Examples abound of older adults who create works of art, start second careers, learn new skills—and maintain their physical health and fitness. Our cowriter, journalist John Hanc, has written many stories about individuals in their seventies and eighties who are (just to use some of his profile subjects of the past year or two) successful composers, writers, historians, professors, fundraisers, and coaches.

They're living, breathing examples of the brain's ability to continue to adapt and learn well into their lives.

The takeaway: don't think your brain cannot respond to stimulus or training because you are now a certain age.

It *can* and it *will*—if you challenge it. As I have seen in my practice, this is achievable even by older adults who already have been compromised by early stage dementia.

Their brains, too, have plasticity. Their brains, too, can adapt.

Recognition of that adaptive ability is one of the most striking and important changes in our understanding of the brain since I've been a neurologist. While I jokingly cavil about having had to take the recertification exam, the truth is that it's thrilling to see the broader context of the science behind what I do daily. And the implications, particularly as we consider brain and heart health together, are enormous.

In the next chapter, we'll look at how we can make that happen.

CHAPTER 2

Lessons of Lifestyle in the Fight against Cardiovascular Disease and Alzheimer's Disease

---

A **COMMON BOND EXISTS BETWEEN** your heartbeats and brain waves that ties their fates together. We know, for example, that people who suffer from congestive heart failure are at a much higher risk of loss of brain function. It is also quite common for someone who is diagnosed with the condition known as atherosclerosis—clogging and hardening of the arteries—to progress to dementia. Even a disruption within the body's tiniest blood vessels can cause significant disturbance to the blood-brain barrier and impair the ability of both organs to operate at full capacity. (This is particularly important for females, as many women experience arterial contraction in small blood vessels, thereby restricting blood flow, as opposed to men, who typically have plaque in larger coronary arteries.)

What's behind the connection? Blood flow is certainly part of it, but there's a lot more to the emerging heart-brain connection: we now know that the well-known risk factors for cardiovascular disease are very similar to those of Alzheimer's disease. Both hypertension and type 2 diabetes, for example, long known as culprits for cardiovascular disease, are also risk factors for Alzheimer's disease. Recent research suggests that ApoE4, the genetic signature associated with higher rates of Alzheimer's, is also implicated in heart disease. In addition, elevated cholesterol—again, a well-known risk factor for heart disease—is linked to higher levels of amyloid, the substance that forms the brain tangles that are a hallmark of Alzheimer's.

The relationship gets broader and deeper: Stroke, high blood pressure, overconsumption of unhealthy fats, excess body weight, smoking, lack of exercise—all well-known cardiovascular risk factors—are now linked to Alzheimer's as well.

This means that we have the power to prevent these diseases and to improve our overall health in the process. *That's* the uplifting promise and purpose of this book.

Yet for years, plenty of learned skeptics were convinced that no matter how virtuously you ate or how many hours you dedicated to the treadmill, the brain and heart would inevitably march toward deterioration. (Truth be told, some still feel this way.)

The idea that a healthy lifestyle could have a positive impact on one's heart health, much less one's brain and heart health together, was a foreign concept in 1977, when Joe Piscatella began to pick up the pieces of his life after his coronary bypass at age thirty-two.

JOE'S JOURNEY: AN EDUCATION FROM THE HEART

"Joe Piscatella knows more about healthy living and the health impact of our lifestyle choices than anyone I know," said Dr. William C. Roberts, MD, director of Baylor University's Heart and Vascular Institute.

I was deeply moved by this endorsement. Dr. Roberts is an eminent and widely respected figure in cardiac medicine, and the fact that he recognizes my hard-earned knowledge about heart disease and prevention—as does the National Institutes of Health, for whom I served as the only nonmedical member of their Cardiac Rehabilitation Expert Panel, charged with developing clinical guidelines for physicians—is both humbling and gratifying.

You could say that what I learned about the heart and cardiovascular system was a form of compulsory education, as it began when I faced a stark reality about my own mortality.

But back in 1977, at the time of my heart surgery, I knew little more than your average person about the heart—and even less about coronary heart disease. What did blocked arteries or heart attacks have to do with me? After all, I was just thirty-two years old and in the prime of my life. There was plenty of time, I thought, to read all those American Heart Association pamphlets while I was rocking in retirement.

I was wrong. Indeed, what I didn't know not only could have hurt me; it could have killed me—and very nearly did.

What I didn't know as a young professional climbing my way up the ladder and raising a family in postwar America was that coronary heart disease develops silently and insidiously over a long period of time, generally twenty to forty years. In my case, it had probably been gradually occluding my arteries for years. Once it surfaces, however, the results—angina, stroke, and heart attack—are devastating.

What I didn't know was that over 4 million Americans had coronary heart disease and that some 1.5 million a year suffered heart attacks resulting in more than five hundred thousand fatalities.

What I didn't know was that two people die every sixty seconds in the United States from some form of heart disease.

What I didn't know was that heart disease causes almost half of all deaths in the United States each year—more than cancer, auto accidents, floods, and airplane disasters combined—and that for 50 percent of all heart-attack victims, their first heart attack resulted in death.

And to cap it off, what I didn't know at the time was that lifestyle, the way we choose to live, was the most important factor in increasing or decreasing cardiac risk.

As I discovered, many if not most in the medical community were equally in the dark about the importance of *what* we do, as opposed to *who* we are, when it came to heart disease prevention and treatment. In fact, I'm not sure how many physicians in that era even thought about prevention. They were trained to recognize what happened when things were going awry, which they were doing with enormous frequency in those days. While it remains the number-one killer in America, the number of deaths from heart disease was significantly greater back then according to the CDC. I think a large part of that is because of what we've learned about prevention.

It all changed for me after July of 1977, when I had coronary bypass surgery. I then became intensely interested in my heart and my heart disease. I remember at the time reading a magazine article about El Cordobés, the famous Spanish matador, who said that his interest in the bullfight increased in direct ratio to the closeness of the bull's horns.

That's it! I thought. That's the approach I'm going to take with this. I put on my metaphorical cape and decided to enter the ring, determined to get so close to the horns of my health dilemma that I could feel their lethal sharpness.

What helped speed me along my journey was my interaction with an eminent cardiologist when I asked for his help. You see, in 1977, not a lot was known about cholesterol, so it was hard to get straight information. But I was lucky, I thought, that a lipid clinic, designed to study cholesterol, had just opened in Seattle. The eminent cardiologist was hired to run the program. "That's it!" I said to my wife, Bernie. "I'll go through the program, meet with the famous doctor for his recommendations, and then our lives will get back to normal."

About eight weeks after my surgery, my primary cardiologist suggested I meet with the lipid specialist. When I sat down in his office, he barely looked up at me. "Mr. Piscatella," he said out loud as he flipped through my charts. "I see you had bypass surgery for coronary artery disease. How are you feeling?"

"Better. Thank you, Doctor," I said. "But I have some questions."

"About your procedure?"

"No," I said. "My question is about what I can do now that the surgery is over. I'd like to know what I can do to help prevent this from happening again."

He raised an eyebrow.

"Well, there might be some medication, and you'll see your cardiologist here for regular checkups," he said.

"Of course," I said. "But I was thinking beyond that. What about things I'm doing in my life? About my diet, about . . . exercise? About my job? Should I be thinking about changing the way I live?"

"Mr. Piscatella," he said. "You're thirty-two years old. You have aggressive coronary artery disease. To be frank, I doubt you'll live to forty."

I imagine my jaw must have dropped—at least slightly. But he wasn't done.

"I see here," he continued, looking at my paperwork, "you have two children?"

"That's right," I said. "Anne is six, Joe is four."

He paused.

"I'm sorry to tell you, Mr. Piscatella, but I think you should face the facts," he said. "If you think you'll live to see those two kids graduate high school, it's probably not going to happen."

More than forty years later, I still shake my head as I recall this conversation. I should add that in the many years since that day, I've worked with researchers and physicians who are just as or more qualified as that gentleman—and who were far more open-minded, not to mention tactful and sensitive in their discussions with patients.

"So, Doctor," I continued, "you're saying that there's *nothing* I can do?"

"I'm not a big believer in exercise and diet," he said. "I'm a believer in DNA and family history. And yours, quite frankly, is not good."

He did have a point there: we have a history of high cholesterol on my mother's side. My maternal grandfather died in his early fifties of a heart attack, as did a cousin. My cholesterol was between 275 and 300, although no one had seemed too concerned about that before I had the chest pains.

"As much as it pains me to tell you this, I think it's important to be honest. This is not going to end well for you," he said.

When I got home that night, I related the story to Bernie. "He said you're going to be dead by the time you're forty?" she said. "Well . . . *that's* not an option. Giving up and just waiting for a . . . a premature death is definitely *not* an option. Listen, Joe. You can't change the cards you were dealt, but you can change the way you play them. I don't care about the nonadvice you just received. We are going to eat better, exercise more regularly, and manage our stress. We are going to create a heart-healthy lifestyle to even up the odds."

Bernie was right. In her own way, she described what science was finding: that cardiovascular health encompasses two basic components. The first is ideal health factors—things like blood pressure, cholesterol, and weight. The other is ideal health behaviors such as non-smoking, eating a healthy diet, and exercising regularly. The latter became my focus.

I vowed to go all in on my El Cordobés approach. I decided to systematically and seriously research this. I would learn as much as I could about how the way we lived, ate, exercised, and managed our lives might be able to improve my heart health—and keep me alive at least a few years longer.

These were the days before you could just Google "heart disease prevention" and have precisely 565 million hits in

0.80 seconds (as I did just now). Doing this kind of research in the late 1970s meant going to a library—and not just the public library, where books for general audiences on heart health were still few and far between. I decided to go to the University of Washington Medical Library.

I informed my primary cardiologist of my intention, and he knew well enough not to try to dissuade me—in fact, I think he sensed I might be on to something.

Off I went to Seattle. The university's Health Sciences Library was an impressive building. I walked in wearing street clothes and found myself surrounded by mostly men in scrubs or white coats. These were the physicians and medical students who were doing research in the library. They were residents, fellows, professors.

I walked up to the front desk and introduced myself. "I'd like to learn more about cholesterol," I said haltingly to the librarian.

"Certainly," she said and returned with several books. Odd, I thought. It was almost as if she was expecting me. I later learned my cardiologist had called the library and forewarned them that a patient of his would-be visiting them soon.

I took the books, sat down, took out my pen and note-book, and started reading.

Five years later, I wrote my first book on how to successfully manage heart disease through lifestyle.

That's a pretty good gauge as to how productive my time in that library, and others, ended up being. As research will, my initial readings in the University of Washington Medical School Library sent me scurrying in new directions. The difference at first was that I wasn't writing an article or a paper or—at that point—a book. I was learning what I could about heart disease in order to put what I learned into action in my own home.

Soon, I was sharing with Bernie what I'd been learning. It wasn't all just from medical journals, which, at the time, were beginning to seriously look at the role of lifestyle in the nation's number-one killer through such already established and important ongoing research as the Framingham Heart Study in Massachusetts.

I also began to look at popular literature, particularly when it came to the details of diet and exercise. *Runner's World* magazine, for example, was a fairly new publication then, and it was filled with articles about people who had improved their heart health through running. I was inspired reading about these fit-looking ex-smokers who were now crossing the finish line of the Boston Marathon. I went out and bought a pair of the still-new Nike "waffle bottom" shoes and began walking, and soon jogging, around the lake near our house. In a few months, I was up to five miles. I swear, the first time I completed that distance nonstop, I felt like I'd won a gold medal in the Olympics!

Meanwhile, books and magazine articles about "heart-healthy" eating (a new term then) were starting to appear. Bernie and I began reading and scouring recipes. My wife is a wonderful cook, and she has a good eye for looking at a recipe, knowing what to take out and add (in fact, Bernie would contribute 250 recipes to my first book—no mean feat!).

At the time, super-low-fat diets were just being introduced. But she and I realized that nobody will eat healthy food that doesn't taste good. So we started creating healthy alternatives that were still appetizing to both us and our kids. Up to that time, we'd eaten like most Americans: cheeseburgers, roast beef, steak, and fried chicken were typical dinners. Not anymore. Over those months in late 1977 and through 1978, we began eating more fish and more fruits and vegetables—all the things that we know now are good for preventing heart disease. Back then, it was still new, however. I'd come home from work, and Bernie would have fixed, say, halibut three different ways—all of which were delicious. Heck, I'd never even tasted halibut before my heart surgery! Ditto with yogurt. Not only did we start eating it, but we made our own low-fat variety. We also made our own mayonnaise with safflower oil. It tasted rich—and delicious! (This was before heart-healthy versions of common foods were available.)

We were looking for every kind of edge. Our education didn't come solely through reading either. Bernie and I attended lectures about heart health that were starting to pop up. I recall driving several hours into Northern California to attend a presentation on some of the latest research. The culture was changing; medicine was changing. Research was beginning to show that with exercise and diet, Americans could fight back against the self-created scourge of heart disease—not necessarily with drugs but by changing their lifestyles.

This we were certainly doing—and it began to show. In the first few months of my new dietary and exercise regimen, I lost ten pounds, I had more energy, and I slept better. Most importantly, my numbers began to go down. Back then, they didn't look at ratios or triglycerides, but as I recall, my total cholesterol went down about forty points, as did my blood pressure. And as they say these days, I "crushed" the treadmill test (conducted then on a massive, creaky treadmill at the local lab, unlike the sleek variety found in gyms today).

While my cardiologist had been very supportive of my effort to change my lifestyle, he expressed concern about me running long distances. "Five miles?" he said incredulously when I called him to tell him about my big achievement. "That's a long way, Joe. I think it's great that you're out walking, but I hope you're not planning to run that far on a regular basis." While he was in favor of my increased physical activity, vigorous exercise was still considered by some to be dangerous for heart patients. But he saw my progress, saw my numbers get better, saw how I looked, and heard how I felt. I knew I'd passed some kind of crucial milestone the night he called me to ask where he could get a pair of running shoes for himself.

Almost five decades later, I'm still exercising. Bernie and I follow a similar diet, and we've made many other adjustments along the way, as more and more research has confirmed what only a few suspected in 1977—how you live your life has an enormous effect on your heart health.

What's so exciting for me today is that these so-called lifestyle interventions—now established dogma in heart disease prevention, treatment, and management—are being shown to have similar beneficial effects on our brains as well.

DR. SABBAGH: THE HEART-BRAIN-LIFESTYLE CONNECTION

Joe's story is so inspiring. It reminds us that when it comes to our health, it's not just medications, surgeries, or genetics that determine outcomes. To a large degree, we call the shots based on what we do.

We know (and Joe has been a pioneer in this area) that the right actions can reverse heart disease. That's well established. But what can these behaviors—these "lifestyle interventions," as we call them in medicine—do to improve our brain health and possibly forestall or prevent Alzheimer's disease and other forms of dementia? If we still adhered to the old, immutable brain model that we discussed in the last chapter, the answer would be *nothing*. There's *nothing* you can really do for brain health—except maybe avoid getting repetitively pounded in the head, like a boxer. That's what I was taught as a young neurology student.

But as we've learned more about the active, plastic brain, we've also learned that there are things that can most definitely help. However, the evidence on these lifestyle factors in brain health is relatively new and still a little less conclusive in some areas than in heart health.

So here's my short answer to the question of whether eating right, exercising, and doing some of the other things we talk about in this book can play an important role in brain health: yes, it can.

To better understand how and why, let's look at one of the bigger research breakthroughs in my field in the past few decades. As *Science Daily* put it in a 2018 article, "Mounting clinical and epidemiological evidence has pointed to a link between heart disease and Alzheimer's disease. Many patients diagnosed with Alzheimer's disease also show signs of cardiovascular disease, and postmortem studies reveal that the brains of many Alzheimer's patients show signs of vascular disease, which some scientists speculate could drive the onset of dementia."

This connection between heart disease and Alzheimer's disease was a bombshell when it first emerged. As the link became better understood, the hope among some was that we could somehow prevent Alzheimer's by treating cardiovascular symptoms with medication. But clinical trials of statins to treat Alzheimer's disease proved largely ineffective. At some point, we may very well be able to do it with medication. But at present, at least for those in the early phases of Alzheimer's, there is evidence that we can push back against the disease with something else.

There are some caveats to that, but generally, the research is now showing that many of the same lifestyle interventions that can help for a healthy heart can also work for a healthy brain. Just what are these behaviors? The Cleveland Clinic's Healthybrains.org lists six ways to improve brain health. Get moving, eat smart, control risks, rest well, keep sharp, and stay connected.

I daresay these are more or less identical to what Joe and others in the cardiac health community would suggest. As you will read later, there are other lifestyle interventions that go beyond the standard recommendations and that are proving useful as well.

But I think it's important for the readers of this book—looking at the connection between heart and brain health—to get a little more granular here. I'd like to share with you the results of a few interesting studies done in the last decade that give us the confidence to make these recommendations.

The first study, published in the journal *Neurology* in July 2020, is particularly fascinating because it uses data from the long-running Framingham Heart Study (something Joe was reading about back in the 1970s as he got himself educated on heart disease and prevention). The study establishes connections between lifestyle and brain health, finding that good cardiovascular health can cut dementia risk in *half*. That's huge.

In the study, researchers examined cardiovascular health data and dementia screenings from 1,211 participants in the Framingham Heart Study. The participants were then scored based on the American Heart Association's seven components of cardiovascular health: physical activity, cholesterol, healthy diet, blood pressure, weight, blood glucose, and smoking status.

The team found that participants with a favorable cardiovascular health score were *55 percent* less likely to develop dementia than participants with an unfavorable score.

There was another interesting variable investigated in that same study: it was found that participants with a high genetic risk score based on several common gene variants were 2.6 times more likely to develop dementia than participants with a low genetic risk score. The researchers, most of whom were from Boston University, also looked separately at the dementia-associated ApoE4 genotype, which is found in 10 to 15 percent of the general population, and found that those with at least one ApoE4 allele were 2.3 times more likely to develop dementia than participants without one.

More about ApoE in a moment. But here's the really interesting part of what they learned in this aspect of their investigation. The researchers found no interaction between genetic risk score and ApoE4 and cardiovascular health, suggesting that these risk factors were independent. This meant that if you had the higher-risk gene variant but practiced heart-healthy behaviors, your risk of getting dementia was *still* more than half.

In other words, nurture trumped nature. What you did mattered more than what you inherited from your parents and grandparents.

My colleague Dr. Sunsar Seshardi, who was one of the investigators on that study and founding director of the Glenn Biggs Institute for Alzheimer's and Neurodegenerative Diseases at the University of Texas Health Science Center at San Antonio, put it well: "We have long maintained that genetics is not destiny, that the impact of your family history and genetic risk can be lowered by healthy lifestyle choices. This is true for persons with low genetic risk and also for persons with high genetic risk of dementia, so it is never too soon and never too late to adopt a heart-healthy lifestyle."

We know now that such a heart-healthy lifestyle is also good for your brain.

BLOOD FLOW AND BEYOND

And the answer is . . . blood flow.

That might seem to be the obvious response to the question of why researchers are seeing this emerging and growing connection between heart and brain health.

While the answer is partially right, it's incomplete. As we said earlier, having a strong heart and sharp mind involves more than blood flow. Optimal heart and brain function involve a complex and multifaceted relationship between many aspects of our cardiovascular and neurological systems. Much of the evidence in this area relates to the link between cardiovascular risk factors and Alzheimer's disease. We think, for a smart reader like yourself, it would be valuable to understand some of this as we go forward with a good program to develop good heart and brain health together.

While not an all-inclusive list, here are some important ways in which conditions generally associated with heart health are now understood to affect brain health as well.

Hypertension

Every time you go in for a checkup, your blood pressure is checked. With good reason—the American Heart Association lists no fewer than seven serious threats related to unchecked hypertension. High blood pressure can result in heart attack (because arteries can become blocked). High blood pressure can result in stroke (because the blood vessels in the brain can become blocked). But high blood pressure can also have other unwanted and dangerous effects: it can cause erectile dysfunction in men, lower libido in women, vision loss, and angina.

Clearly, there are lots of good reasons to keep your blood pressure at normal levels! But researchers are now discovering even more. One 2019 study found that treating high blood pressure reduced dementia risk by 12 percent and the risk of developing Alzheimer's disease by 16 percent. While medication was used to lower blood pressure in that study, we know that a healthy lifestyle—exercise, diet, and stress reduction—can help manage hypertension. According to the Mayo Clinic, "Lifestyle plays an important role in treating your high blood pressure. If you successfully control your blood pressure with a healthy lifestyle, you might avoid, delay or reduce the need for medication."

The Clinic offers a list of ten lifestyle measures that are effective in achieving that goal (https://www.mayoclinic .org/diseases-conditions/high-blood-pressure/in-depth/ high-blood-pressure/art-20046974). Perhaps not surprisingly, that list is consistent with the steps we advocated for brain health: diet, exercise, weight management, smoking cessation, and so on.

Taking these steps can help lower hypertension, which, in turn, can lower your risk of dementia and help keep your brain, as well as your heart, healthy.

Why? Because hypertension causes a thickening of the walls of the blood vessels. Smaller vessels mean less blood circulation, especially to the deep parts of the brain that are responsible for cognition, memory, and executive function. Over time, it is theorized, this may lead to actual changes in the brain, some of which could be the kind of pathology we see in Alzheimer's—including atrophy of the cortex and the infamous plaques and tangles that are a hallmark of the disease.

Homocysteine

While you've likely heard of hypertension, it's doubtful that you were checked for your homocysteine levels during your most recent physical.

Homocysteine is a blood protein—a by-product of normal metabolic activity. But we know that when it's elevated, you can have an increased risk of heart attack, stroke, *and* dementia.

Red meat consumption is associated with higher levels of homocysteine. But just cutting back on your burgers and steak is probably not sufficient. The way you reduce homocysteine is by taking B vitamin supplements—specifically, B_9, the synthetic form of folic acid.

Yes, as opposed to the many misleading or downright false claims made about the benefits of supplements, this is one area where they are warranted. We'll discuss that further in our nutrition chapter, but suffice it to say for now that homocysteine is another good example of the convergence of heart and brain health and how they can be impacted by something within our control.

Cholesterol

As Joe told us earlier in this chapter, even back in the 1970s, high cholesterol levels were known to be associated with heart disease. Like your blood pressure (and unlike your homocysteine level!) cholesterol work-ups have become a common part of any blood test.

Your physician is mostly looking at your levels and ratios with a view toward your heart health. But in the past decade, we've become aware that managing one's lipid profile could be critical to brain health as well. A 2020 review of over one hundred studies found that elevated cholesterol is indeed a risk factor for Alzheimer's disease (https://doi.org/10.3390/brainsci10060386).

However, the research paints a more nuanced picture. All forms of cholesterol are not created equal, at least when it comes to their effects on our brain health. Total cholesterol, triglycerides, and high-density lipoproteins (HDLs, the so-called good cholesterol) were *not* implicated in Alzheimer's disease. But high levels of low-density lipoproteins—LDLs, also known as "bad" cholesterol—lived up to their billing. It was elevated levels of this form of cholesterol that were most closely associated with Alzheimer's.

Moreover, some of the studies examined in this meta-analysis showed that elevated LDLs in midlife increases the risk of developing Alzheimer's in later years—perhaps not surprising given the long, gradual progression of the disease.

While the pathway for how this happens and why LDLs as opposed to HDLs or total cholesterol might be involved in the onset of Alzheimer's remains unclear, that finding is a clarion call to action: if you can take steps now to reduce your LDL, you may be helping lower the risk of developing Alzheimer's later.

And what's one of the best ways to lower LDL? Yes, it's lifestyle.

ApoE

If you're looking for a "smoking gun" in the mystery of the heart-brain connection, ApoE might be it.

When this genetic interrelation was first discovered in 1993 (during a heart-related study about lipids, by the way), researchers found that carriers of a variant of this gene had a higher lifetime risk for developing Alzheimer's disease. And if you have *two* copies of the gene—one from each side of the family—your risk of getting the disease can be as high as 91 percent (as was the case with Alzheimer's advocate Jamie Tyrone, with whom John Hanc and I collaborated for a 2018 book, *Fighting for My Life*).

However, before we start treating ApoE like a film villain, we must recognize that the picture is more complex. ApoE is not out to get you. As part of the metabolic process, it's actually designed to *help* you. ApoE provides instructions for making a protein called apolipoprotein E. This protein combines with fats (lipids) in the body to form molecules called lipoproteins, which are responsible for packaging cholesterol and other fats and then transporting them through the bloodstream, where they can then help prevent various disorders affecting the heart and blood vessels (yes, it seems that cholesterol—at normal levels—is not all bad either!)

There are three different "alleles" (or versions) of the ApoE gene, known as E2, E3, and E4. The most common is E3, which is found in 80 percent of the population and doesn't appear to affect the risk of either heart disease *or* Alzheimer's disease.

E2, the least common variant, can be considered a mixed blessing to the estimated 5 percent of those who have it: while ApoE2 may increase the risk *for* heart disease, it can actually protect *against* Alzheimer's.

That leaves E4, another culprit in heart disease. This variant can significantly increase levels of harmful LDL cholesterol and triglycerides. In fact, carriers of an E4 allele are at a 43 percent higher risk for coronary heart disease. But E4's potentially adverse health effects don't stop there: dozens of studies have confirmed that its presence increases the risk of developing age-related cognitive decline and Alzheimer's disease. In fact, it's estimated that up to 60 percent of all people with late-onset Alzheimer's disease are ApoE4 carriers. While we are not sure why, we do know that when ApoE4 lipoproteins bind to cell-surface receptors to deliver lipids, it causes connections between brain cells to start to break down—the same kind of degeneration we see in cases of Alzheimer's.

In that sense, ApoE4 stands guilty as charged: research has implicated it as a genetic risk factor in *both* heart disease and Alzheimer's disease.

But let's stop for a moment and consider this word: *genetic*. I've noticed that when people hear this uttered—when, for example, I explain to patients and families that their loved one's condition has a "genetic" basis—they tend to throw up their hands, thinking it's all beyond their control. We can't possibly do anything to alter this predetermined fate, right? It would be as futile as trying to change your eye color or the texture of your hair. So why bother?

But, as I remind my patients, that is *not* the case with many things related to their health—and certainly not with the gene variant so closely associated with both Alzheimer's and heart disease. As the Mayo Clinic points out in a 2019 article on ApoE4, not everyone who has this variant of the gene develops Alzheimer's. And many who get the disease *don't* have the gene. This suggests that ApoE4 is a risk but not a cause and certainly not a fait accompli when it comes to getting Alzheimer's—or heart disease, for that matter.

What's more, even if you *do* have the ApoE4 gene, your behavior can offset its potential effects. Genetics is not necessarily destiny, as one of the world's largest studies on senile dementia has shown:

As part of the Finnish Geriatric Intervention Study to Prevent Cognitive Impairment and Disability (FINGER), a randomized controlled trial conducted at several sites in Finland, over 1,100 older adults (with an average age of 69.3 years) were randomly assigned to a group that made lifestyle changes or a control group that just received general health advice. Of this large group, 362 participants had at least one copy of the ApoE4 allele.

After two years, ApoE4 carriers who made the lifestyle changes had improved overall cognitive function and memory when compared to carriers in the control group. It's also interesting to note that those *without* the ApoE4 gene who made the lifestyle changes appeared to improve on cognitive functions too, though this effect was not statistically different when compared to those in the control group.

And what were the lifestyle modifications that produced these encouraging results in that 2018 study? The very same ones advocated by many champions for brain health and by many major health institutions.

Forty years ago, as you've read, the idea that someone with heart disease could change his fate by changing his lifestyle would have been scoffed at by some. Joe Piscatella proved the skeptics wrong—and over the years, he has inspired thousands of others to do the same. I believe that we are at the point when Alzheimer's and other forms of senile dementia can be viewed in the same way.

You can't change your genes, but you can change your life. Let's get started.

CHAPTER 3

Your Scorecard for
Heart and Brain Health

HELPING READERS ACHIEVE OPTIMAL heart-brain health while keeping heart disease and Alzheimer's disease at bay is the goal of this book. How do you measure your progress along the way? By establishing critical markers.

In this chapter, Joe Piscatella will provide a "vital signs" scorecard—assessing the most important values for heart-brain health. Some of these will be familiar, such as high-density lipoproteins (HDL) and low-density lipoproteins (LDL). But as there is clear evidence now about the link between hypercholesterolemia and cognitive disorders, we move into more sophisticated values—particle size and apoproteins.

Similarly, we drill down into other values and look at measurements related to cognitive health and how these can be gauged.

The goal here is not to get you to run off and schedule a battery of additional tests beyond the ones you should be having as part of routine medical screenings. But as the association among things like metabolic syndrome, inflammation, stroke, type 2 diabetes, and both heart disease and Alzheimer's disease becomes clear—a link that we discussed in the previous chapter—it's important to be aware of these benchmarks.

To get some of your numbers, you may need to check the results of your most recent blood test. Many physicians will send these to you after a blood work-up as part of a routine physical, but if you don't have them, you can probably call your doctor's office to get a copy. And remember, many of these risk factors—levels of physical activity, for example—are easy to gauge and track.

Now let's go over the risk factors and scorecard with Joe.

"IF YOU DON'T KNOW WHERE YOU ARE GOING, YOU MIGHT NOT KNOW WHEN YOU GET THERE"

That classic Yoga Berra axiom applies to both heart and brain health. Let me speak to cardiac health as an example. Although we often focus on cholesterol and its role in heart disease, in reality, there are a number of critical factors that work individually and in concert to produce the disease and, conversely, produce heart health. Historically, the coronary arteries have been described as akin to PVC "pipes." Should cholesterol accumulate as plaque and block the pipes, blood flow to the heart is slowed or stopped, often resulting in a heart attack. This is an easily understood concept, but it is too simplistic an explanation. The fact is that there are some 250 cardiac risk factors, some of which—such as inflammation—rank right up there with cholesterol.

So suddenly cholesterol is only one in a group of interrelated factors that together play a causal role in a heart attack. In other words, you should know your cholesterol numbers. But you should also know where you stand with other key critical risk factors as well.

That's the reason for the scorecard. Recognizing that not all cardiac risk factors are of the same weight, we've identified eleven key factors such as blood pressure and weight. By knowing the numbers—*your numbers*—for each key risk factor, you can identify where you are now and, perhaps more importantly, where you need to be to optimize heart (and brain) health.

Here is an example. The National Cholesterol Education Program has issued a recommendation that triglycerides be "below 150 mg/dl" to qualify as a "desirable risk." But let's suppose your triglycerides are 300. You know what your triglyceride score is, and you can then take action—such as losing weight, exercising regularly, and reducing refined sugar consumption—to reach the "desirable" goal.

That is the reason for creating the scorecard—to give you a starting point for health factors critical for heart and brain health and a goal of where you want to be. Later in the book, we explain what actions can be taken to reach your goals.

It is also important to understand that cardiac health markers tend to cluster and "feed" on one another. Multiple factors do not simply add to your risk. Instead, there is a geometric progression that increases heart-attack risk with each additional factor. The Framingham Heart Study, the oldest heart study in the country (and referenced in some of the research we discussed in the previous chapter), found that if you only have one factor—let's say you smoke or you have high cholesterol or high blood pressure—you have twice the risk of heart disease as someone without any of these markers. But if you have two of the three markers, your risk quadruples. And if you have all three, your risk is *eight* times greater.

The way that risk factors come together to become greater than the sum of their parts is why we have identified eleven total factors. Start by examining your numbers to create a profile of where you are now. Some of your numbers may be well within your goals. If that's the case, keep on doing what you are doing. But if they are short of your goals, go to work to improve them.

The good news is that changing lifestyle habits can improve your numbers—and your health—immensely. Harvard's Dr. JoAnn Manson conducted a study on some eighty-five thousand women. She found that lifestyle changes, even moderate ones, produced multiple risk reductions, culminating in a 31 percent drop in heart disease over fourteen years. The findings were so clear that Dr. Manson was able to calculate the reduction in cardiac risk from specific lifestyle changes.

Behavior	Reduction in Heart-Attack Risk
Stop smoking	50 percent to 70 percent lower risk within five years of quitting
Reduce blood cholesterol	1 percent reduction in cholesterol produces a 2 percent to 3 percent drop in risk
Manage high blood pressure	1 mm Hg reduction in diastolic pressure produces a 2 percent to 3 percent drop in risk
Exercise regularly	Active lifestyle reduces risk by 45 percent
Maintain ideal weight	Results in 35 percent to 55 percent lower risk, compared with those who are obese

Seattle cardiologist Steve Yarnall explains the situation this way: "You don't have to be a scientist to understand that the grease you sandblast from your oven and soak off your dishes isn't something you want in your arteries. You don't have to be a physiologist to understand that regular, moderate physical activity is preferable to no exercise. And you don't have to be a genius to figure out that setting fire to tobacco leaves and inhaling smoke doesn't make a whole lot of sense."

One last important point: you learned in the last chapter about the powerful connection between cardiac risk and cognitive problems; between cardiovascular disease and Alzheimer's disease. We've identified in this chapter some measures that are commonly and easily gauged by either you or your physician. Cognitive testing is more typically done by a neurologist, such as Dr. Sabbagh. But later in this book, he will offer some thoughts on how you can develop criteria to assess the brain part of the heart-brain health equation.

Chances are, if you follow the scorecard here, your brain health will already be improved by the time you read that section!

1. BLOOD PRESSURE

Blood pressure is the force needed to move blood through the vascular system in the body against the resistance of artery walls. Think of an ordinary garden hose. The water pressure decreases when the nozzle is opened. But pressure is increased if the nozzle is closed.

High blood pressure, or hypertension, is usually caused by a narrowing of arteries and arterioles or a lack of elasticity. These conditions create resistance, which in turn creates pressure, causing the heart to work harder pumping blood throughout the system. One potential result is an aneurysm, the bulging and rupture of an artery, stroke, hardening of the arteries, heart attack, kidney failure, congestive heart failure, and death. High blood pressure can also cause inflammation of the coronary arteries, which is a trigger for heart attack.

Some sixty-three million Americans, mostly of middle age, suffer from high blood pressure. It is more common in African Americans than in other races. High blood pressure is responsible for forty-five thousand deaths each year in the United States and contributes to the deaths of an additional 210,000 people. People with high blood pressure are up to five times more likely to have a heart attack and more than twice as likely to have a stroke as people with normal blood pressure. Ironically, according to American Heart Association estimates, over 50 percent of American adults with high blood pressure don't even know they have the condition.

Blood pressure usually progresses silently, increasing year after year. Often symptoms earlier in life can seem benign, such as dizziness, swelling in the ankles and feet, headaches, changes in vision, and leg cramps. Then suddenly in middle age, hypertension appears. Unfortunately, by this time, it is often too late to repair any damage done such as type 2 diabetes and macular degeneration.

Blood Pressure Scorecard

Blood pressure is expressed as two numbers representing millimeters of mercury (mm Hg). Systolic pressure, the top number, is taken when the heart beats, the moment when blood is pumped out of the heart in one big burst of peak pressure and the aorta expands to handle the flow. Diastolic pressure, the bottom number, is registered between heartbeats when the pressure falls to its lowest point. This is when the heart relaxes, regains its normal size, and refills with blood. Normal systolic pressure is 120 mm Hg and normal diastolic pressure is 80 mm Hg, typically recorded as 120/80 and expressed as "120 over 80."

Historically, it was felt that diastolic pressure was more important. That's because this number reflected the minimum pressure to which the arteries are constantly exposed. As such, it was found to be less variable than systolic pressure. Today, however, that thinking has changed. Both numbers are used to diagnose the presence and severity of hypertension.

The following standards have been established by the National Institutes of Health for assessing high blood pressure. You should use this information on your scorecard.

Blood Pressure Reading

Systolic	Diastolic	Risk
Below 120 and	Below 80	Normal
120 to 139 or	80 to 89	Prehypertension
140 to 159 or	90 to 99	Stage 1 hypertension
160 and above or	100 and above	Stage 2 hypertension
Your systolic pressure: _____		Your diastolic pressure: _____

It is very important to check your blood pressure regularly. If your readings are usually within normal range, keep on doing what you are doing. But if they're consistently out of the normal range, take action by using the prescriptive measures in this book to help you lose weight, moderate salt intake, and become more physically active.

2. TOTAL CHOLESTEROL

Nothing is more closely identified with heart disease and heart attacks than cholesterol—and rightly so. When there is too much cholesterol in the blood, it tends to clump together on the inner walls of coronary arteries, clog the channel, and prevent blood from reaching the heart. It is for this reason that high cholesterol is cited as a major culprit in coronary heart disease. Still, cholesterol is not the be-all and end-all of heart disease, nor is it toxic. It occurs naturally as a soft, waxy substance in all cells. In truth, cholesterol is not all bad. Essential for cell wall construction, the transmission of nerve impulses, and the synthesis of important hormones, it has a legitimate role in the healthy functioning of the body and poses few problems when present in the correct amount. When levels in the blood are excessive, however, cholesterol can accumulate on the coronary artery walls.

It is an acknowledged axiom that the higher the level of blood cholesterol, the greater the risk of heart attack. But just as increased cholesterol levels can cause the incidence of heart attack to rise, decreased levels have been shown to cause heart-attack incidences to drop. Indeed, numerous studies have illustrated that for every 1 percent reduction in total cholesterol, there is a 2 percent reduction in cardiac risk. At first glance, this may not seem significant. But the disease may progress at a rate of 2 percent to 4 percent a year when cholesterol stays high, so the net gain from lowering cholesterol may be as much as 6 percent a year. Dr. William C. Roberts, editor-in-chief of the *American Journal of Cardiology*, states that whatever your total cholesterol is, reducing that number by about forty points cuts your risk of a heart attack in half.

While reducing cholesterol can produce coronary regression (reversal) in some people, newer studies focus on plaque stabilization. This is important because unstable plaque can rupture, spill cholesterol into the bloodstream, and produce a clot that can trigger a heart attack. Lowering cholesterol tends to stabilize plaque and reduce cardiac risk.

While concern over the years has been on total cholesterol, today it is critical to look at the factors that make up that total number, specifically LDL and HDL cholesterol. All three cholesterol numbers are a part of your scorecard.

Total Cholesterol Scorecard

Cholesterol levels are easily calculated from a blood test. The results are expressed as the number of milligrams (mg) of cholesterol per deciliter (dl) of blood. For example, the level of a person who has 200 mg of cholesterol in a deciliter of blood would be 200 mg/dl, simply expressed as "200."

You and your doctor can't determine your cardiac risk or formulate a response strategy unless you know your cholesterol number. The National Cholesterol Education Program, in collaboration with the American Heart Association and other medical authorities, has issued guidelines for total cholesterol.

Total Cholesterol	Risk Classification
Below 200	Desirable
200 to 239	Borderline high
240 and above	High
Your number: _____ Your risk: _____	

Heart patients and those who have two or more risk factors should strive for a level no higher than 200, preferably in the 150 to 160 range.

3. LDL CHOLESTEROL

In the case of cholesterol, the whole is less important than the sum of its major parts: low-density and high-density lipoproteins (LDL and HDL, respectively).

Studies show LDL to be an independent risk factor for coronary heart disease. The higher your LDL, the greater the cardiac risk.

Predominantly made of fat and very little protein, LDL transports about 60 percent to 80 percent of the body's cholesterol through the bloodstream. Circulating in the blood for several days after its creation, LDL is taken up by body cells as building blocks for hormones and cell parts. But the cells may not require all the cholesterol that is delivered. The excess floats in the blood, collects on artery walls, causes inflammation, and creates plaque. This is why LDL is commonly called "bad" cholesterol.

LDL Cholesterol Scorecard

The National Cholesterol Education Program created the following scale to assess cardiac risk from LDL.

LDL Cholesterol	Risk Classification
Below 100	Optimal
100 to 129	Near optimal
130 to 159	Borderline high
160 to 189	High
190 and above	Very high
Your number: _____ Your risk: _____	

4. HDL CHOLESTEROL

High-density lipoprotein, called HDL, is known as "good" cholesterol because it doesn't form plaque. Furthermore, it acts as a scavenger, picks up excessive LDL from artery walls, and transports it to the liver for removal from the body. Because HDL helps prevent cholesterol from building up on the walls of the arteries, a high HDL level is considered cardioprotective.

While HDL averages only about 25 percent of total cholesterol, it is critically important. Low HDL, defined as below 40 for men and below 50 for women, is considered a predictive risk factor. A high level of HDL, defined as 60 or higher, is associated with lower risk. It is estimated that for every 1 mg increase in HDL, there is a 4 percent decrease in cardiac risk.

HDL Cholesterol Scorecard

The National Cholesterol Education Program created the following scale to assess cardiac risk from HDL.

HDL Cholesterol	Risk Classification
60 and above	Low
40 to 59	Moderate
Below 40	High
Your number: _____ Your risk: _____	

5. TRIGLYCERIDES

Most of the fat in your body is in the form of triglycerides. Calories consumed during a meal and not used immediately are converted into triglycerides and transported to fat cells, where they are stored for energy. However, a small portion is found in the bloodstream as a component of lipoproteins. At normal levels, triglycerides play a positive role in good health. But numerous studies have shown that elevated triglycerides are a risk for coronary heart disease, heart attack, and stroke, particularly in women who are overweight, hypertensive, and diabetic. In addition, high triglycerides are often accompanied by other risk factors, such as high blood pressure and low HDL. The bundling of these factors is reflected in a cardiac marker called metabolic syndrome, which can have serious cardiac consequences.

Triglyceride Scorecard

Measured by a blood test, triglycerides are expressed as the number of milligrams on one deciliter of blood. The normal range is 50 to 150, depending on age and gender, but being overweight and obese, physical inactivity, smoking, excess alcohol intake, high-carbohydrate diets, several diseases (such as type 2 diabetes), certain drugs (such as higher doses of beta-blockers), various genetic disorders, and liver and kidney disease all contribute to elevated triglycerides.

The American Heart Association recommends keeping your triglycerides below 150 mg/dl and, if possible, under 100. The Adult Treatment Panel III Guidelines suggest these risk classifications:

Triglycerides	Risk Classification
Below 150	Desirable
150 to 199	Borderline high
200 to 499	High
500 and above	Very high
Your number: _____	Your risk: _____

6. METABOLIC SYNDROME

Metabolic syndrome is actually a cluster of cardiac risk factors: abdominal obesity, high triglycerides, low HDL level, elevated glucose, and high blood pressure. Each of these symptoms is a significant risk in its own right; however, in combination, the sum of the parts creates an even greater risk. People with metabolic syndrome are twice as likely to have a heart attack and three times as likely to develop diabetes.

Because people with this condition typically have a moderate level of total cholesterol, often under 200, metabolic syndrome may be overlooked in a medical exam. For example, data on a fifty-one-year-old male in the Framingham Heart Study produced the following lipid profile:

Total cholesterol	195
LDL cholesterol	108
HDL cholesterol	32
Triglycerides	264

It might be assumed that because his total cholesterol was under 200 and his LDL was "near optimal," this man had a low cardiac risk. In fact, the man had coronary heart disease that was likely attributable to metabolic syndrome. Says Dr. William Castelli, "In Framingham, we found that when triglycerides are high and HDL is low, the predictive risk of heart attack doubles . . . even when total cholesterol is in line. We also found that when you fatten up in the abdomen, you start to move your triglycerides and HDL toward metabolic syndrome. And when you add in high blood pressure and diabetes, the effect is disastrous."

Metabolic Syndrome Scorecard

The American Heart Association / National Heart, Lung, and Blood Institute published the following risk profile for metabolic syndrome:

Is your HDL below 40 (men) or below 50 (women)?	Yes _____ No _____
Is your triglyceride number over 150?	Yes _____ No _____
Is your waist size 35 inches or above (women) or 40 inches and above (men)?	Yes _____ No _____
Is your blood pressure consistently 130/85 or greater?	Yes _____ No _____
Are you a prediabetic or diabetic (a fasting glucose of 100 or greater)?	Yes _____ No _____

If you answered "yes" to two of the five questions, you probably have metabolic syndrome.

If you answered "yes" to three or more, you *definitely* have metabolic syndrome.

(Note: Recognize that the answer to HDL, triglycerides, blood pressure, and fasting glucose questions should be "yes" if you are taking medication to correct them.)

7. WEIGHT

Carrying too much weight is linked to a variety of diseases and debilitating conditions such as elevated cholesterol and high blood pressure. Compared with people of normal weight, obese people have a 50 percent to 100 percent greater risk of premature death. For example, an eight-year study of 110,000 American women aged thirty to fifty-five showed that those as little as 5 percent overweight were 30 percent more likely than their lean counterparts to develop heart disease. That risk increased to 80 percent in women who were moderately overweight, while those who were obese were more than 300 percent more likely to develop heart disease.

Despite these connections being well understood by the public, the American waistline continues to expand. Nearly 70 percent of the adult population is either overweight or obese. No nation in the history of the world has experienced the obesity problem of modern America. Indeed, the typical man weighs twenty to thirty-plus pounds too much, and the typical woman is overweight by fifteen to thirty-plus pounds. To make matters worse, surveys show that nearly 82 percent of Americans gain weight every year. While it is tempting to blame genetics, research suggests that what we weigh is largely determined by our environment and how we live. Ours is a fast-food, overeating, couch-potato, video-game culture that makes it all too easy to put on extra pounds.

Consider the impact of our national weight problem:

- Experts warn that obesity and physical inactivity may soon surpass smoking as the nation's principal cause of preventable death.
- Actuarial studies have found that the death rate from all causes increases as weight rises, particularly for obese people weighing 30 percent or more above ideal weight.
- "Five of the 10 leading causes of death in the U.S. are linked to weight," says cardiologist Dr. Charles H. Hennekens of the University of Miami Medical School.

Weight Scorecard

The National Institutes of Health recommends using the body mass index (BMI) to assess your risk. BMI describes body weight relative to height. Here is a BMI table. To use the table, find your height in the left-hand column labeled "Height." Move across to your weight. The number at the top of the column is the BMI value for your height and weight.

BMI*	Condition	Risk
19 to 24.9	Healthy weight	Desirable
25 to 29.9	Overweight	Borderline high
30 to 39.9	Obese	High
40 or above	Very obese	Very high
Your number: _____	Your risk: _____	

* BMI usually correlates well with body fat, although very muscular people may have a high BMI without excess body fat. In that case, there is little or no added health risk.

8. ABDOMINAL OBESITY

The link between overweight and heart disease is particularly strong if the excess weight is carried in the abdomen. Says Dr. William Castelli, former director of the Framingham Heart Study, "People with wide hips and flat bellies may be overweight, but the extra weight does not seem to increase their cardiac risk as much as that of people with narrow hips and potbellies. Such abdominal obesity is predictive of cardiac risk."

Potbellies make people, mostly men, appear "apple-shaped," while other people, mostly women, could be described as "pear-shaped." Perhaps because abdominal fat is more metabolically active than fat stored in thighs, hips, and buttocks, "apples" are three to five times more likely than "pears" to suffer heart attacks.

Are you an "apple" or a "pear"? You can determine this simply by measuring your waist. The American Heart Association defines a high-risk waistline as thirty-five inches or more for women and forty inches or more for men.

Abdominal Obesity Scorecard

Waist Circumference	Risk Classification
Men	
Less than 40 inches*	Lower
40 inches and above	Higher

Waist Circumference	Risk Classification
Women	
Less than 35 inches*	Lower
35 inches and above	Higher
Your number: _____	Your risk: _____

9. GLUCOSE

Glucose, or blood sugar, is used by the body for energy. Insulin, a hormone produced by the pancreas, is necessary for the body to absorb glucose. But in the twenty-four million Americans with diabetes (some 8 percent of the population), the body does not produce insulin (or produces too little of it) or the body does not properly use the insulin that is produced. As a consequence, glucose builds up in the blood and eventually begins to appear in the urine. Over time, high glucose levels can cause stroke, high blood pressure, blindness, kidney disease, nerve damage, and amputation.

Diabetes is the fourth leading cause of death in the United States. Type 2 diabetes, the form most commonly linked to cardiovascular disease, is the number-one cause of death. It usually strikes people in their forties or older and accounts for 90 percent to 95 percent of all diabetic cases. About one-third of the people with type 2 diabetes do not know that they have it. Although there seems to be a genetic predisposition in some people—particularly African American,

Hispanic/Latino, Asian American, Pacific Islander, and Native American populations—most type 2 diabetes is triggered by obesity. Indeed, more than 85 percent of the type 2 diabetes population is overweight or obese.

It is important to know your risk for diabetes, particularly if you have a family history. Experts recommend that all adults over age forty-five be tested for diabetes every three years with a fasting glucose test. The results of the fasting glucose test are represented as milligrams of glucose in one deciliter of blood. The American Diabetes Association suggests that the following scale be used to estimate risk:

Glucose Scorecard

Glucose	Risk
Below 100	Normal
100 to 125	Prediabetes
126 or higher	Confirmed diabetes
Your number: _____ Your risk: _____	

If your glucose level is even slightly elevated (100 to 125, for example), a blood test called hemoglobin A1c is suggested. A1c measures the amount of glucose attached to red blood cells. The higher your blood glucose, the more sugar will accumulate in your red blood cells over time. Because red blood cells live 90 to 120 days, this test reveals your "average" blood sugar during that time. For people without diabetes, target A1c numbers range from 4 percent to 6 percent. Those with diabetes or coronary and other vascular diseases should strive for a value below 7 percent. In investment terms, knowing your blood glucose level is akin to checking where you are today with your stock portfolio. A1c is like checking your portfolio for the quarter.

10. HOMOCYSTEINE

Remember the skinned knee you had as a child? Remember how it turned red and felt hot to the touch? That's because white blood cells congregated at the site of the wound. The proteins that were then released to enable the wound to heal produced inflammation that lasted until healing was underway.

It's the same with injuries to coronary arteries. These arteries flex and twist each time the heart beats, causing minute fissures in the artery lining. Since the heart beats more than one hundred thousand times a day, there is nothing we can do about these wear-and-tear injuries, all of which may cause inflammation. Genetic makeup can also produce arterial injuries. For example, some people have high levels of an amino acid called homocysteine in their blood, which, in excess, can damage artery walls. And finally, certain factors (hypertension, elevated LDL cholesterol, diabetes) and lifestyle habits promote arterial inflammation. Each time a smoker inhales, nicotine and carbon monoxide are released into the bloodstream, irritating the artery walls. Stress, which can cause adrenaline and other powerful hormones to race through the blood vessel system, can also cause injury.

The danger here is that chronic inflammation destabilizes plaque, which allows cholesterol to enter the bloodstream and form a clot, which can stanch blood flow to the heart and brain. As Harvard Medical School researcher Dr. Paul Ridker says, "We have learned that coronary heart disease is very much an inflammatory disease, the same way that arthritis and lupus are inflammatory diseases." The implications are enormous. Dr. Ridker estimates that between twenty-five and thirty-five million healthy, middle-aged Americans have normal cholesterol but above-average inflammation, putting them at risk of heart attacks and strokes.

A good way to estimate your inflammatory response is to check your homocysteine levels. When you eat meat or vegetable proteins, your body initiates a series of biochemical reactions that ultimately lead to the production of homocysteine. In proper amounts, homocysteine in the blood is not a health threat. But an inadequate dietary intake of the B vitamins (especially folate) or certain genetic defects can elevate homocysteine levels.

High homocysteine damages the linings of blood vessels, triggering the growth of cells that form the framework of plaque. It also promotes the breakdown of LDL cholesterol within the plaque, which can lead to blood clots. At one time, experts speculated that high homocysteine was not the cause of arterial damage but the result of damage already done. If that were the case, then reducing homocysteine in the blood would not provide any coronary protection. Newer research suggests the opposite conclusion: lowering homocysteine may reduce cardiac risk.

The exact process by which high levels of homocysteine contribute to coronary heart disease is not fully known. About 20 percent to 40 percent of people with coronary heart disease have elevated homocysteine.

At present, there are no professional guidelines to determine who should be tested for elevated homocysteine. Most doctors test patients who have had a heart attack, bypass surgery or other signs of heart disease, or a strong family history. But because it is such a strong marker, many physicians are now screening for homocysteine as part of a standard lipid panel.

Homocysteine is determined with a blood test called Abbott Homocysteine, which describes your level as the number of micromoles per liter of blood (umol/l). Experts consider 5 to 15 umol/l to be a normal range, although heart disease risk begins to rise at 9. As the level of this marker goes up, so does the likelihood of heart disease.

Homocysteine Scorecard

Homocysteine Level	Risk
Less than 5	Desirable
5 to 9	Normal
10 to 30	Moderate
31 to 100	High
Above 100	Severe
Your number: _____ Your risk: _____	

11. PHYSICAL ACTIVITY

Like blood pressure and cholesterol, your level of physical activity is another part of your score.

Why is that? you might wonder. Exercise is something you do—it's not something you are. Yet how much activity we engineer into our lives—whether it's counted in minutes, miles, or steps—is now seen as closely linked with heart health (and increasingly, brain health) that it has to be included as part of any baseline health calculation.

While there is unanimity in the medical community that we should be exercising, how we go about it is a different question. What type of exercise is best? For how long should it be done? And at what intensity level? There are so many views about the best way to get active, from so many different expert groups, it's sometimes hard to know what provides the most sweat equity.

And of particular importance to this book: Are there exercise regimens that can actually promote both heart and brain health together?

The answer to that last question is a resounding yes!

Exercise is such an important part of the strong heart–sharp mind formula that we've devoted an entire chapter to it in this book. A fair chunk of that chapter addresses the so-called exercise prescription—meaning the correct "dose" or amount of physical activity needed to accrue its many benefits.

For the purposes of this scorecard, you can use the current national physical activity guidelines released by the

Health and Human Services Department in 2018. Their exercise prescription is mirrored by most major public health organizations, including the National Institutes of Health, the American Heart Association, and the Centers for Disease Control and Prevention.

Here's what they advise: "For health benefits, adults should do at least 150 minutes (2 hours, 30 minutes) a week of moderate-intensity activity or 75 minutes (1 hour, 15 minutes) a week of vigorous-intensity aerobic activity."

Physical Activity Level Scorecard

Activity Level	Risk Classification
150 minutes or more of moderate-intensity activity	Lower
75 minutes or more of vigorous-intensity activity	Lower
Less than 150 minutes of moderate-intensity activity	Higher
Less than 75 minutes of vigorous-intensity activity	Higher

Just a quick note of clarification as you're putting together your scorecard. One hundred and fifty minutes may sound like a lot, but when you average it out over the course of a week, we're talking about a brisk thirty-minute walk five days a week. If you're not already doing that, you should be—and you *can* be, as it's hardly an onerous time commitment. And if you'd rather push the pace and follow the more vigorous intensity standard, the time commitment is even less: three sessions of less than a half hour weekly.

YOUR RISK PROFILE

Now that you have the information on individual cardiac risk factors, it's time to tally them all up. We're keeping it simple. Go back to the eleven risk factors and see where you stand based on the values you know. Are you high risk or low risk? Are you at optimal levels or is this is an area where you need to do some work?

Risk Factors	Is This a Risk for You?	
	Yes	No
1. Blood pressure		
2. Total cholesterol		
3. LDL cholesterol		
4. HDL cholesterol		
5. Triglycerides		
6. Metabolic syndrome		
7. Weight		
8. Abdominal obesity		
9. Glucose		
10. Homocysteine		
11. Physical activity		

How did you do? If you have nine or more factors that do not constitute a risk—if, say, your blood pressure is in line and your cholesterol levels are where they should be—good for you! Continue doing what you are doing. But if you have factors that constitute a risk for you—perhaps your triglycerides are too high?—then it's time to take action on lifestyle habits that can reduce that risk (in the case of elevated triglycerides, cutting sugar consumption and losing a few pounds.)

Remember, risk factors are real, but so are the effects of positive lifestyle habits. In the next chapters, we'll explain how to use those habits to manage heart and brain risk factors and guide you through a program that can help with both. At the end of this book, you can come back, revisit the risk factor scorecard, and get a perfect eleven!

CHAPTER 4

They Did It—So Can You!

Profiles in Heart-Brain Health

WE'VE DISCUSSED THE SCIENCE behind the heart-brain connection and its importance as a nexus of health. We've provided you with a scorecard of values to help you in your journey toward optimal health.

In the upcoming chapters, we provide an overview of our evidence-based plan toward achieving this goal, which involves some surprising new twists on familiar behaviors. For example, we recommend the following:

- Exercise, *but* with a new combination of activities—including some suggested workouts—designed to maximize the heart-brain connection.
- The Mediterranean diet, *but* with a fresh look at the recently revised dietary pyramid and a few specific

new suggestions for heart- and brain-healthy nutrients, informed by the most recent research.

- Stress management, *but* with the recommendation of a new technique that has been shown to calm the body and brain in only twelve minutes and help improve cognitive function, to boot.

We do the same with the other components of our six-step program—plus new iterations and twists—that you can follow and incorporate into your lifestyle. Each chapter will also include a motivational, first-person perspective from Joe Piscatella and a closer look at the science with Dr. Sabbagh as well as actionable tips and advice.

In this chapter, we start by offering you two case studies of individuals who have successfully followed programs similar to the one we offer in this book. These people are just a few of the many who have made massive overhauls in the way they live their lives and are now feeling better and healthier than they ever have. You might need similar modifications in the way you live your life—or you may only need to make some tweaks. Either way, we think you'll find the stories of these people motivational: One of them is a patient of Dr. Sabbagh's who came concerned about memory loss and left with a prescription for brain- and heart-healthy lifestyle changes. The other case study follows a husband and wife who Joe Piscatella first met on a drizzly, overcast evening a few years ago outside of Seattle.

CASE STUDY: JOE PISCATELLA

How Playing the Cards You're Dealt Can Make All the Difference

I stood off to the side of the stage at the Lynnwood Convention Center and watched as the audience filed in to take their seats.

It was a typical early spring evening in Washington state—damp and overcast: a weeknight where a more appealing option might have been to stay home, put your feet up in front of the TV, and munch on potato chips. Then again, I reflected, for many of those in attendance that night, it might have been a little too much of that sedentary behavior and junk food consumption that had compelled them to show up in the first place.

We were here in this Seattle suburb to kick off the third annual edition of 6 Weeks to a Healthier You with Joe Piscatella. Our program was organized in conjunction with the Verdant Health Commission, a local public health organization that had advertised my program as an opportunity for local residents to "create the foundation for developing new healthy lifestyle habits."

Many of those residents were now filling up the auditorium at the Convention Center. More than half in attendance were female, and the average age was around fifty. But beyond that, there was very little homogeneity in this audience. They came in all shapes and sizes and from all walks of life. The growing sea of individuals that settled into their seats before me, I learned, ranged from professors at nearby Edmonds Community College to guys who pumped gas at the Shell Station off Route 405. We had computer scientists from Microsoft, assembly-line workers from Boeing, office workers from the Lynnwood Corporate Center, and cashiers and clerks from Nordstrom and JCPenney at the Alderwood Mall.

While I certainly realize that income disparities are linked to health and that folks in prosperous suburbs like Lynnwood have distinct advantages over those in poor rural communities or inner cities when it comes to access to health care, observing the diversity of the audience that night reminded me of how democratic and accessible personal health behaviors can be. If you're willing to put in the work, you can reap the benefits, regardless of who you are or what you do for a living.

That was essentially the premise of our event: anyone interested in making changes to improve their heart health was welcome to come.

And they did. By 6 p.m., the vast, 1,200-seat auditorium was over two-thirds full.

After a representative from Verdant welcomed everyone, I walked out and took my place behind the lectern, flanked by two huge screens that displayed my Power-Point slides on healthy eating, stress management, and exercise.

"Good evening, everyone," I said. "I'm Joe Piscatella." I offered them one of my stock lines: "I like to say that you can't control the deck of cards you're dealt, but you can control how you play them. And that's what we're going to show you how to do, starting tonight."

*   *   *

As we related in the last chapter, my writing career began seven years after my bypass surgery, in 1982, with the publication of *Don't Eat Your Heart Out*, a book that went on to sell over a million copies. I gave advice on how to live a heart-healthy lifestyle, and my wife, Bernie, contributed over 250 delicious yet healthy recipes.

In the following years, more books were written on healthy eating, effective exercise, stress management, and developing a positive mind-set. Soon I was giving some eighty-five lectures a year to medical professionals, patients, companies, associations, and the general public. I even sat on a National Institutes of Health Expert Panel that developed clinical practice guidelines for physicians—heady stuff for a nonmedical person.

Soon my information found its way to three PBS television specials on heart health that I hosted and to a column on WebMD.

While the acceptance of my work was much appreciated, it felt incomplete. After all, I was writing and speaking on lifestyle changes, but so far, I only had one test case: me! I was doing extremely well in my postbypass life, but I felt a little guilty that I had only obtained data from one person. I was painting a picture of how to live a healthy lifestyle for thousands of people but had no granular data to back it up.

That's when I had an idea to put together a motivational educational program that would help people improve their heart health in six weeks based on my personal experience and research. Week one was healthy eating, week two was exercise, and so on. There was even a week for a cooking demonstration and another for raising fit children.

After a few trial programs with great results (in one Michigan program, 650 people lost a total of 4,200 pounds), we were ready to face a larger audience over a long period.

And that's how I ended up in Lynnwood, staring out at a sea of faces.

The program consisted of me delivering sixty- to ninety-minute talks, self-scoring tests (such as "Are You a Type A Personality?"), and homework (walking for fifteen minutes and eating oatmeal for breakfast). The talks were laced with stories, anecdotes, and personal observations. Even my failures were discussed. For example, in the stress session, I related how I once received two speeding tickets in twenty minutes (just for the record, the first ticket made me late!).

Everybody registered in the program received testing for biometric measurements including weight (BMI), blood pressure, cholesterol, LDL, HDL, triglycerides, and glucose as well as questions on exercise and stress. This testing took place prior to the 6 Week program and after the program as well. This would allow me to see if my healthy lifestyle theories worked for more than just me.

"Know Your Numbers" was the title of my first slide—a reminder to this audience of why we had them get tested (and consistent with what we addressed in the previous chapter of this book: the importance of having a scorecard of values to gauge your progress by.)

Since my healthy living information was always seen through the prism of cardiac health, it was no surprise that many in the audience had specific problems—high cholesterol, high blood pressure, excess weight.

In the audience that night were a husband and wife who could check "yes" after every one of the risk factors: James and Mary Camino. Both in their early sixties, both obese, both saddled with high cholesterol. At the time they first attended my session, they were also both recently retired: Mary from a local hospital, where she had been a nurse for many years, and James at one of the area high schools, where he'd been a high-school social studies teacher and a baseball coach.

In every person's life there comes a "teachable moment"—an event or experience that presents a good opportunity for learning something about a particular aspect of life. In the case of James and Mary, the teachable moment for making changes in their lifestyle had occurred two years prior to my talk, when James had bypass surgery. He developed complications, and the poor guy had to have his chest reopened two more times by the surgeon. It got worse: as a result of the surgeries, James started to throw clots, which resulted in a massive stroke. He lay in a coma in intensive care at the hospital while on the heart-lung machine and on pulmonary life support. Their daughter flew home from college. Last rites were administered. No one expected him to live.

Meanwhile, Mary could only look on and pray, realizing that many of James's problems—such as weight and cholesterol—were the same ones she faced. Women get heart disease too—in fact, it's the number-one killer among women in the United States. Was this her future too?

Like many in that situation, Mary's prayers involved bargaining with God: "If you let my husband live," she said through clenched hands and closed eyes, "we'll both clean up our acts, I promise."

In this case, the Almighty apparently responded, "Deal." James pulled through. But his quality of life was poor. His mobility was limited. He felt miserable. Mary wasn't much better. She'd quit smoking a few years earlier, but she could barely climb up the stairs from their den to the kitchen. Her doctor was concerned, and she was too. So when she saw the ad Verdant had placed for my seminar, she signed up immediately. "This is exactly what we need," she told James. How excited her husband was initially at the prospect of sitting in an auditorium on a Wednesday night and being told how he had to change the way he'd done things his entire life, I can't say. But I suspect his near-death experience and the fact that, in his present condition, he would be incapable of playing catch with any future grandkids made him a lot more open to the idea of change than he would have been otherwise.

Clearly, they were ready to learn. Ready to make big changes. In fact, that's exactly what he and Mary said during our brief introductions. "We're ready to do what we have to do, Joe," Mary said, earnestly, as we shook hands. James just nodded. Although he said nothing, I do recall sensing a glint of determination in his eye.

Day by day, week by week, the Caminos made a profound transformation in their lifestyle. They did things the way we recommend (and that we'll talk about in each aspect of the program in this book). Start slowly, make changes gradually.

But change they did.

They began by cutting out soft drinks—the Caminos apparently loved their Cokes, but Mary learned to enjoy nonsweetened ice tea, and James found that tonic water, sometimes with a twist of lemon, became his new beverage of choice.

As Bernie and I had many years earlier, they began experimenting with new alternates in the kitchen: the fryer sat unused, there was low-fat frozen yogurt in the freezer instead of ice cream, and the Caminos began discovering how tasty chicken and fish dishes could be (although, no offense to Mary, I can't imagine she's learned to make halibut as delicious as Bernie's!).

Activity is, of course, an important part of our program: the Caminos started walking, at first around the block of their neighborhood because that's as far as either of them could make it. But they continued—here's that word again—*gradually* increasing the distance to the point that they eventually got up to a mile, then a mile and a quarter, then a mile and a half. A few days before the last of our six weekly meetings in the program, the Caminos completed a three-mile hike on the trails of Scriber Lake Park. "Three miles, Joe!" exclaimed an animated James when he saw me at that meeting. "A year ago, I could barely get out of bed. You have no idea how that feels."

Actually, I did. I smiled as James related this to me, recalling the exhilarating feeling I had when I first walked the then inconceivable distance of five miles after my heart surgery.

The Caminos did some of the other things that we recommend as part of a heart-healthy program—they had been through a lot of stress the previous years, principally with James's health problems and some of the financial strains they'd been under, since both were newly retired at the time. Now the couple both tried to take a few minutes each day for some deep breathing. Mary, in fact, began to listen to meditation tapes. Joe discovered the joys of listening to "hot stove" baseball podcasts as he continued his walks on the beautiful trails around Scriber Lake.

Not surprisingly, the Caminos graduated from my program with flying colors. Their numbers were already moving in the right direction after six weeks. But I think what's even more gratifying is the message I received from James recently. Actually, it was from Mary, but she got her husband to sit down at the computer and tap out his part, which I thought was kind of nice: "Hi Joe, I'm still eating healthy and walking four miles a day, at least five days a week. Mary's been taking a Jazzercise class, and sometimes I join her for that as well. So far, I'm down 54 pounds since I first met you. Last week I had a follow-up appointment and my blood pressure was 120/62, and my resting heart rate continued to drop, from 67 to 52."

James went on to tell me that Mary (who also lost significant weight) is off blood pressure meds. Moreover, both of them have had to purchase new wardrobes. "My old pants were just too baggy," he joked. In closing, James wrote, "I just wanted to thank you for the support. My doctor says I've probably added five years to my life."

Not everyone who has attended my seminars has had quite the dramatic turnaround in their lives that James and Mary did, in part because most were not in the dire straits that they had found themselves in a few years ago. Many more needed only to make smaller adjustments to get to where they needed to be.

Still, this was tremendously gratifying to hear. And there was one last thing James told me during our most recent communication that I want to share with you because it relates directly to the premise of this book.

Now that he's feeling better physically, James has gotten back into coaching with one of the local Pop Warner teams. He's also a big Mariners fan and watches with the eye of someone who really knows the game. Like some serious fans, he actually keeps score, which means carefully observing and recording every batter and every pitch. "Joe, it's a funny thing," he said. "After my heart attack, while I was recovering, I had to stop keeping score. I couldn't keep track of things. My brain felt fuzzy. I thought maybe it was just old age, or something to do with the surgery." But now, he says, "I'm as sharp as I ever was, watching a game, and keeping track of it. It's almost like I can think more clearly."

A stronger heart *and* a sharper mind? I think we could say that James now has both—and it was because of the changes he and Mary made in their lifestyles.

CASE STUDY: DR. SABBAGH

How Small Steps Lead to Big Results

Robert trudges into my offices accompanied by his wife, Trish. It is clear that she is the one insisting on this visit. He looks reluctant, sheepish, and a bit guilty.

As if they had agreed to it beforehand, Trish speaks as he sits, staring at the floor. "Dr. Sabbagh," she begins, "he's having trouble concentrating on the job, he says, and I see it at home too. I'll be in the middle of a conversation, and halfway through, he forgets what we we're talking about. He's also tired all the time, he says he can't sleep, but when he finally does get to sleep, there's the snoring . . ."

Robert shrinks into his seat a bit, embarrassed. He would probably prefer it if his wife stopped sharing what he views as personal information, but this is exactly the kind of information I need. Robert, who is fifty-eight at the time of his initial consultation with me, has been referred by his primary, in part because Trish was concerned—and she has every right to be. Her husband, who is sweating and red-faced from either the stress of this visit or his poor health, is visibly obese, and I can only imagine some of the values I'll find when we get his blood work back.

"Robert, Trish was right to have you come see me," I say, addressing him. "Is there anything you want to add? How are you feeling?"

He sighs. "Yeah, I know, she's right," Robert says, grabbing Trish's hand and squeezing it. "Some days I feel like I'm walking around in a fog. I keep thinking it's because I can't sleep, but . . ."

He looks at Trish. "Tell him," she says. "There's nothing to be ashamed of."

Robert furrows his brow. "Well, the truth is, doc, I'm a little worried about Alzheimer's. It runs in my family. I saw my mother go through it, and . . . well, I wouldn't want Trish or the kids to have to deal with that."

"Let's not get ahead of ourselves," I say. "I'm sorry to hear about your mom, but let's take a look at what's going on before we jump to any conclusions."

Upon examination, we find that Robert's BMI is 35—that's almost morbidly obese—and his blood pressure is 170/105. Very high. In addition to some of his other symptoms, he reports occasional chest pain and admits to having fallen asleep in a meeting at work.

I come up with an initial plan: we're going to get Robert into a sleep study—meaning a clinical program that can help identify and address his sleep issues. I'm also going to refer him to a cardiologist and prescribe neuropsychological testing to get a better sense of what's behind these concentration lapses. I also order an MRI.

A few days later, I get the results. The cardiologist's report confirms what I suspected: based on a thorough examination that included an echocardiogram and a treadmill test, the cardiologist diagnoses Robert with ventricular hypertrophy—thickening of the heart wall as a result of his high blood pressure. Based on this, the cardiologist elects to get a cardiac catheterization to locate any blockages and finds that Robert does indeed have stenosis—obstruction—in his arteries, including a worrisome blockage in the left anterior descending artery. That's the infamous "widow maker."

Trish doesn't want to be a widow, I think as I read the results, which is why she was wise to compel her husband to get an examination.

Meanwhile, the sleep study shows that he has moderate-severe obstructive sleep apnea. His blood work reveals a total cholesterol level of 260. His triglycerides are nearly 300, and his waist size is forty inches. His homocysteine levels were also tested. Ideally, we want those lower than 10. Robert's homocysteine levels are twice as high. Additionally, genetic testing reveals that's he's an ApoE3-4, meaning he has one allele from his father and one from his mother.

If we measure these values against the scorecard we presented in the last chapter of this book, Robert is not doing well. But there are a few bright spots. The MRI showed little ischemic white matter change. The deterioration of these deep brain fibers can be a precursor to Alzheimer's, so this is a good sign. Also, his psychological test came up normal. There are no cognitive deficits we can see and, at least for now, no sign of the disease that his mother suffered from.

A few days later, Robert and Trish are back in my office, listening as I go through the results. "Robert, you have multiple risk factors," I say. "But I'm happy to say that I don't see any signs of Alzheimer's."

He sighs with relief. Trish is happy, but she knows there's a "but."

"That's great news, Dr. Sabbagh," she says. "But he's got to make some changes, doesn't he?"

"He does. As I said, Robert, you don't have Alzheimer's now, but that could be exactly what you're looking at in the future."

He seems puzzled. "So it's because of my mom . . . because it runs in the family?"

"That's only a small part of it. You're at risk for Alzheimer's in large part because you're at high risk for coronary artery disease."

Both he and Trish look back blankly at me. I'm not surprised at this reaction: many if not most of my patients are unaware of the link between heart health and brain health.

"Wow," he says. "I had no idea there was a connection."

"But, Doctor," says Trish, who is already a step ahead, "if he could lose weight, like I've been telling him to do for years . . ." (*a sharp glance at her husband*) ". . . and if he could start exercising and eating right, does that mean he could be helping his heart but also be helping prevent Alzheimer's too?"

I tell Trish that while we don't like to use the word *prevent*, she is absolutely right about the positive role lifestyle could play in her husband's brain health. I explain to her what we've learned from some of the same studies I've shared with you in this book. I then address her husband. "Robert," I say, "there are a lot of people with advanced dementia for whom, sadly, there is little that we can do. You're lucky. You've been given an option . . . a second chance."

I urge him to get himself in better condition, change his habits, and bring his numbers down. If he does, his odds of getting what his mother had will be much lower.

But I conclude, "I want to emphasize something here, Robert. Trish can't do this for you, nor can I. We can help, but ultimately, this is up to you."

Robert stares at the floor, nodding, and then looks up and meets my gaze. "I don't want to end up like my mom," he says. "I'll do it." Trish puts her arm around him.

We discuss what this would entail: a comprehensive lifestyle change, including a diet makeover and the implementation of an exercise regimen as well as some other things—for the apnea, a CPAP machine, the idea of which he doesn't like (few do) but agrees to try. He's reluctant to take the cholesterol-lowering medication the cardiologist wants him on, but he does agree to try folic acid supplements and methylfolate, which have been shown to help mood and cognitive function (more about this in our nutrition chapter).

Robert is also willing to try exercise. I want him to start jogging on a treadmill. He will start slow—five miles an hour, or roughly a twelve-minute per mile pace.

"I don't know if I can do that, doc," he says. "The only exercise I've done for the last few years is getting up to go to the refrigerator." Trish rolls her eyes. But Robert quickly adds that he will do his best. "How about if I start by trying to jog for one minute? I know it doesn't sound much, but it's better than nothing, right?"

"I'll take it," I reply, knowing that research has shown that even small amounts of physical activity have benefits. Also, I'd rather Robert starts out with goals that he feels are realistic. But I want to see progression, so I ask him to try to add one minute per week to his jogging intervals.

He agreed. We set a very conservative goal for weight loss as well: two pounds a month. As part of that, Robert also agrees to consult with a nutritionist I refer him to. She puts him on a whole-food, plant-based diet.

Fast forward one year: Robert is back in my office, and he's like a new man in many respects. He's twenty-four pounds lighter, his BMI has gone from 31 to 26, he's lost two inches on his waist, and his blood pressure is down to 140/83. He's up to an hour on the treadmill, his cholesterol has plummeted to 220, and his HDLs have increased significantly.

And although we don't have a metric to measure it, his sleep apnea is much improved, which is improving Trish's quality of life along with the fact that Robert seems more alert—he's no longer nodding out in the middle of meetings or losing track of conversations.

I give Robert a lot of credit—but without Trish push-ing, cajoling, and encouraging him along the way, I wonder whether any of this would have happened. It brings up a few important points.

First, we all need a support system—a little help to make significant lifestyle changes. Very often, I've found that it is wives and mothers who seem to play that role—even though in Alzheimer's, as we know, women tend to have higher incidences (primarily because they have longer life-spans). While some of this may be stereotypical—I've had plenty of male patients who were the driving force for change and female patients who were the ones reluctant to do so—it does say something about those who are determined to take the necessary steps for pos-itive changes in both heart and brain health.

As a reader of this book, I suspect you are such a per-son, regardless of your gender. And while you might not have as far to go or as many habits to change as Robert (or James and Linda, the couple that Joe talked about), you should know that the very act of contem-plating change—as you are doing now—is seen by the-orists as the first and perhaps most fundamental step in making the lifestyle transformations that are going to lead you to the optimal health implied in our title.

There are other aspects of heart-brain health that we will explore. But let's get you going with one of the most important building blocks of the program: phys-ical activity.

CHAPTER 5

Step 1

Functional Fitness for Heart-Brain Health

I N 2008, THE FEDERAL government issued the first national guidelines for physical activity.

Some might joke that they were only twelve thousand years late.

Humans have been physically active since our species first worked up an appetite. The hunter-gatherers we are descended from were engineered for movement. In a fascinating 2012 paper, neuroscientist Mark P. Mattson listed the many ways that this is so, including our long, elastic leg tendons, our sweat glands and sparse body hair, our swivel hips, and—of particular relevance to this book—our advanced cognitive capabilities, which suggest a brain-heart connection that helped distinguish humans from other species and which we contend in this book is now being recognized as a critical nexus of human health.

All these factors helped make us, quite literally, born to run—or at least walk briskly—over long distances. And because we were able to do that, starting about two million years ago and continuing through the end of the hunter-gatherer period, it could be argued that we were eventually able to create civilization.

Early humans didn't need to be told to keep track of their distance in miles, minutes, or steps. And their sojourns weren't just in the pursuit of game. Researchers have speculated that a natural cycle of regular activity, intense and moderate, was likely the norm for most of human existence: one or two days of vigorous and strenuous exertion in the hunt for food punctuated by one or two days of less intense activity, which might have included long walks to nearby villages or to trade with other clans and communities.

This activity pattern—episodes of vigorous and moderate exertion accumulated throughout the day—is not dissimilar to the recommendations made in modern guidelines.

And that's the important point here: the onus on physical activity and exercise, the contemporary fitness culture of marathon running, CrossFit gyms, or Peloton bikes, may seem like a fad, but it's essentially a return to the kind of natural activity that our mind and bodies have been developed for—something that, like language and emotions, is a critical part of what it is to be human.

The Centers for Disease Control and Prevention said as much in a white paper on physical activity in 1999: "Viewed through the perspective of evolutionary time, sedentary existence, possible for great numbers of people only during the last century, represents a transient, unnatural aberration."

In other words, we need to stop thinking about physical activity as something strange, new, and uncomfortable—some kind of castor oil we are being forced to take by people in white lab coats. Rather, we should view it as something that is an inherent part of who we are, a skill or talent you never realized you had. And regardless of how fast or slow your ability to walk, you *do* have this ability. We all do. We've just made it easy for ourselves to forget that by relying on machines to do what our legs or lungs used to accomplish for us.

Of course, no one is suggesting we go back to being hunter-gatherers. So how do we reconnect with the patterns of exercise that are intrinsic to us as humans and accrue the enormous physical and (yes) mental health benefits of exercise?

That's what we will show you in this chapter. And we will go beyond the conventional wisdom that you may have heard. We'll show you why physical activity is good for *both* your heart and your brain—including some interesting new aspects of the fitness equation that can have profound effects on both.

Perhaps most importantly, we'll also show you how

you can start incorporating this into your life and how, in tandem with other essential components of brain/heart health, physical activity can lower your risk of getting both heart disease and Alzheimer's disease (not to mention many other afflictions) and significantly improve the quality of your life.

*   *   *

The 2008 guidelines released by the Health and Human Services Department were updated in 2018 to reflect the latest thinking. The basics, however, are still the same. Here's what they advise: "For health benefits, adults should do at least 150 minutes (2 hours, 30 minutes) a week of moderate-intensity activity or 75 minutes (1 hour, 15 minutes) a week of vigorous-intensity aerobic activity."

It's further recommended that adults should perform muscle-strengthening activities—exercises involving all major muscle groups—two times a week. Older adults should also include balance training.

We'll talk about all of this—and more. But let's underscore some of the guideline's other key points:

Adults should move more and sit less throughout the day. At this writing, many of us have spent weeks indoors because of the COVID-19 pandemic. While necessary to stop the spread of the disease, some public health officials also reminded citizens to get out regularly for socially distanced exercise, even during the lockdown. They knew that long periods of sitting could create its own, slow-burning health crisis. (As one wag put it, "Television can be a weapon of mass destruction." The same could probably be said of the cell phone, the internet, and social media!)

Some physical activity is better than none. Many people still think the only way exercise is going to be effective is if it's long, sustained, and intense. Go out and run or cycle or swim as hard as you can for as long as you can. When you drop to your hands and knees at the finish line gasping for air, you've done what you're supposed to.

No!

That old no-pain, no-gain guideline is a recipe for how to quit or avoid exercising. While vigorous exercise has great value, research over the last few decades has really opened our eyes about the value of what could be called "small" exercise—moderate intensity, shorter duration, especially for those just starting out.

GOT A MINUTE TO TAKE SOME IMPORTANT STEPS FOR YOUR HEALTH?

Epidemiologist Steve Blair, professor emeritus at the University of South Carolina and the former president of the Cooper Institute for Aerobics Research, was a pioneer in establishing the value of short bouts of moderate-intensity activity. Dr. Blair has spoken about the Power of the Two-Minute Walk, which he uses as a rejoinder to those who claim they don't have time for exercise. While two minutes is not sufficient to meet the guidelines, it is enough to surmount the largest hurdle facing most of us when it comes to exercise: simply getting started.

Oh, and just by *doing* that two-minute walk—OK, maybe a couple of times a day—you're already accruing some basic health benefits.

Dr. Blair and the national guidelines talk about minutes, but today, many people like to count steps on a pedometer or an app on their phone. A review of studies in the journal *Medicine & Science in Sports & Exercise* found that about seven thousand to nine thousand steps a day can result in health benefits similar to the federally recommended 150 to 300 weekly minutes.

As for the oft-heard recommendation of ten thousand steps per day, the American College of Sports Medicine offers this tidbit: research supporting the ten thousand steps a day guideline is limited, and some believe the recommendation was actually derived from the name of a Japanese-made pedometer sold in the 1960s called Manpo-kei, which translates to "ten-thousand steps meter."

Should you choose to count steps, which is a convenient and fun way to keep track of your activity, that's fine. So is keeping an eye on the clock as you rack up your federally recommended minutes. And many pedestrians and runners still like to think in terms of miles. After all, there's something satisfying about saying you've walked a mile—or three or five. It makes you feel like you're really going places with your exercise regimen.

Regardless of how you measure it, your goal should be consistent, regular activity, which has innumerable benefits for both your heart and your brain.

Let's examine those more closely now.

EXERCISE: GOOD FOR YOUR HEART

When physicians and public health officials talk about the health benefits of physical activity exercise, they're largely—although not exclusively—referring to its effects on the heart and cardiovascular system. They are significant, as exercise can do the following:

- reduce the risk of heart attack and stroke (The Harvard Alumni Study and the Nurses' Health Study both found that about three hours a week of walking reduced heart-attack risk by 35 to 40 percent.)
- strengthen the cardiac muscle, thereby reducing strain when the heart pumps
- increase HDL cholesterol, which is protective for heart health (A study at Stanford found that walking two miles three days a week would raise HDL by 10 percent.)

- reduce coronary inflammation and blood clotting
- prevent the development of high blood pressure
- build muscle and bone strength as well as balance
- serve as a key to weight loss and weight control by burning calories, elevating metabolism, building muscle, and helping manage stress

It usually takes about three months of consistent activity to achieve these cardio-protective benefits. We'll talk about the "fitness formula" to help you get there a little later in this chapter, but first, here's how one man—Joe Piscatella, coauthor of this book and a nationally recognized expert on heart health—used exercise to transform his own life.

A NEW LIFE THROUGH EXERCISE: JOE'S JOURNEY

I was always an athlete, playing sports in high school and college. But in those days, once graduated, married, and with children, a lot of us just stopped. Oh, there was social tennis and golf, but aerobic exercise wasn't part of my routine. Both my weight and my cholesterol went up.

After undergoing coronary bypass surgery at age thirty-two, the alarm clock of reality rang. On one hand, I had a young family, with children who were just six and four. On the other hand, I had a doctor tell me that because I was so young and the disease so aggressive, I probably would not live to age forty. As my wife, Bernie, stated, "That is not an option!"

So I began my journey to discover how lifestyle habits could impact my heart health positively. Obviously, not smoking (I was a nonsmoker) and eating a healthy diet were priorities, as were managing stress and developing a positive attitude. But for me, exercise became the starting point.

At that time, however, there was a curious dichotomy. The running boom was starting to take off with the general public, but heart patients were told to "take it easy." Many were put to bed. After researching exercise and the potential for cardio benefits, I decided to start running. My doctor went through the roof. "You can't do that," he said. "It will put too much strain on your heart. I forbid it!"

I responded that the last time I checked, it was *my* heart, and so it would be my decision. Clad in an early edition of Nikes, cotton running socks, and (short) running shorts, I began my treks around the neighborhood, eventually running four miles five days a week. Six months later, I was in my doctor's office for a follow-up exam. All of my biometric numbers—cholesterol, weight, and blood pressure—were excellent, and my doctor was well pleased. That evening as we were seated at the dinner table, the phone rang.

It was my doctor with a simple question: "Joe, where do you get your running shoes?"

I ran for the next thirty-plus years until orthopedic problems in my sixties turned me into a brisk walker. Now I walk five miles a day six days a week. My biometric numbers are still excellent.

Three things have kept me motivated over all these years. Initially, I exercised faithfully because of my young family. I did it for them . . . and me. I didn't want to miss my son's graduation from college, walking my daughter down the aisle at her wedding, or growing old with Bernie. As much as we could, we made exercise a family affair. The kids would often join me on my run.

As time went on and my heart health became more secure, I was lucky enough to find excellent exercise partners to keep me committed, on track, and accountable. And I did the same for them. Here is an example. I exercise early in the morning. Up at 5 o'clock, by 5:15 I'm laced up and out the door. This past February, the weather here in the Pacific Northwest was terrible. As my radio alarm went off, I could hear the driving rain pelt the windows horizontally. The radio announcer told me it was thirty-eight degrees, and I was under a down comforter.

I'm not going, I thought to myself. *Who would go out on a day like today? I'm staying in bed.* Then I realized that I have a training partner. I can't call him at 5 a.m. just to say I don't want to walk. So I got up, got dressed, met him at the corner, and off we went. I was glad that we had done it after it was over, but I never would have done it without my exercise partner.

And finally, I have found exercise to be motivating for other aspects of my life, such as eating healthy, managing stress, and thinking positively. For me, exercising regularly forms a foundation of success that allows me to build on my other lifestyle habits.

Throughout my life, exercise has been as natural as brushing my teeth. Once you get into it, it takes on a life of its own.

EXERCISE: GOOD FOR YOUR HEAD TOO!

By the time Joe began his comeback from bypass surgery in the 1970s, the link between exercise and a healthy heart was well established. But it is only in the last twenty years or so that researchers have discovered the many ways physical activity can help our mental and brain health too. These include the following:

- stress management
- mood enhancement
- improved self-esteem
- reduction in anxiety and depression
- better sleep
- improved memory
- greater levels of creativity

Regular exercise, said the Harvard Health Letter in 2018, "has a unique capacity to exhilarate and relax, to provide stimulation and calm, to counter depression and dissipate stress."

"A walking brain is a more active brain," wrote neuroscientist Shane O'Mara in a recent *Wall Street Journal* column, praising this most basic form of physical activity. "Walk we must and walk we should."

You would think, then, that most people—particularly those facing cognitive decline and senile dementia—would embrace physical activity. But that is not often the case, notes the coauthor of this book, neurologist Marwan Sabbagh, MD.

DR. SABBAGH ON EXERCISE AND DEMENTIA: FINGER, EXERT, AND THE BDNF FACTOR

I am still surprised by how deeply sedentary behavior is ingrained in many of my patients' lives. When I encourage them to start walking or to try yoga or a senior aerobics class, they roll their eyes. "Yeah, yeah," they say. "We've heard this."

What they *haven't* heard is how this can help the condition I'm trying to treat as their neurologist. They don't equate exercise with having a beneficial effect on the health of their brain. When I start speaking about exercise in relation to their brain health, they sometimes assume I'm talking about doing crossword puzzles. Yes, that's good, I tell them. But those kinds of cognitive-stimulation exercises—which we'll address in a separate chapter in this book—are different from physical activity and have a different effect.

We know from a number of studies that regular physical activity may be one of the most important things you can do to promote brain health. For example, we know that cognition—which is essentially all aspects of thinking (memory, concentration, language, processing speed, and so on)—improves up to 10 to 20 percent after a structured program is implemented.

We also know that exercise has the potential to reduce the risk of developing dementia. The two-year study known as FINGER (Finnish Geriatric Intervention Study to Prevent Cognitive Impairment and Disability) examined healthy lifestyle interventions among 1,109 people in Finland, aged 60 to 77, who had genetic risk factors for memory disorders. Researchers at the Karolinska Institute looked at diet, cognitive training, and some other interventions that we'll discuss in other chapters of this book. But one of the most striking findings from this investigation was the importance of exercise.

Participants in the study engaged in the kind of structured, multifaceted exercise program we are recommending in this book, including aerobic and balance training for the heart and brain. The results: regardless of their genetic risk, the subjects in the study improved in all cognitive domains, including the speed with which they could process information and their ability to perform complex memory tasks.

Another important investigation, known as the EXERT study, looks at the value of exercise in adults with memory problems. This national eighteen-month clinical trial is testing whether physical exercise—aerobic training, or stretching and balance exercise—can slow the progression of mild memory loss and/or mild cognitive impairment in older people. One of the test sites is the Cleveland Clinic Lou Ruvo Center for Brain Health in Las Vegas, Nevada. As the Center's former director, I can tell you we're excited to be part of this nationwide investigation, the results of which so far are promising and may lead us one step closer to the point where we can, as an NPR story about the EXERT study described it, prescribe exercise as a drug to forestall or prevent Alzheimer's disease.

Wouldn't that be marvelous?

But we already know enough to be convinced of the one-two punch of exercise in heart and brain health. One reason exercise has such a powerful effect is that it promotes blood flow from the heart to the brain—the intersection that, as we say in this book, represents an important new dimension of overall health. But there are other reasons too: Exercise can help reduce or avoid such conditions as hypertension, hyperlipidemia, and diabetes, all of which have been associated with dementia development—again, showing how improvements in the heart and cardiovascular system can often be linked to brain health.

Studies have also shown that, in those who exercise, the volume of the hippocampus—the brain's memory center—is increased and that exercise is key to the production of something called the brain-derived neurotrophic factor, or BDNF. It has also been referred to, in more pungent terms, as fertilizer for your brain.

Here's the science behind it: your brain, like every other part of the body, has the ability to regenerate itself. These growth and healing (also known as *trophic*) agents, or factors, are a family of proteins. They include NGF (nerve growth factor), HGF (human growth factor), and BDNF, which have been linked to improved learning and memory, elevated mood, and the ability to acquire new skills. BDNF has also been associated with lower levels of certain types of inflammation, and there is evidence that those with higher levels of BDNF have lower rates of Alzheimer's disease and dementia.

As the National Medical Library describes it, BDNF is active in cell-to-cell communications, helping regulate what is called "synaptic plasticity"—meaning that it helps the synapses (the nerve endings that connect the neurons of the brain) adapt and change over time in response to experience.

It is nothing less than nourishment for the brain.

So how do you get more of this nourishment? Contrary to the claims of some supplement marketers, you can't take BDNF in a pill. You can't sprinkle it on your Wheaties either. But what you can do is exercise. Because we know that, unlike some of the other growth factors, BDNF production is stimulated by as little as thirty minutes of vigorous exercise three times a week. But even greater gains, writes exercise physiologist Louise Pontin, have been found when you combine that with a more complex activity, which requires you to build or acquire a skill—exercise that challenges your balance or thinking.

And that's the kind of exercise we're going to look at now.

EXERCISE AT THE NEXUS OF HEART AND BRAIN HEALTH

A group of twenty-five older adults at the Linwood Senior Center in Wichita, Kansas, are standing on three-inch-thick foam pads, each of them holding a yellow whiffle ball.

"I'd like you to hold the ball in one hand and then drop it into the other," says the class leader, Dr. Michael Rogers, an exercise physiologist at Wichita State University, as he begins releasing his own ball from the fingers of his right hand into the palm of his left.

The class follows his lead. "Now expand the distance," he says, raising one arm and, thus, the distance that the ball must fall. "Change hands."

Arms swing up and down, brows furrow, and a few balls go rolling on the floor to titters of laughter. As the balls are collected, Dr. Rogers directs their attention to an image projected on the wall of the rec room.

"OK," he says. "I'd like you to read the words."

"Red. Green. Yellow. Blue," the group says in unison, still while standing on the unstable surface the foot cushions provide as they read a series of words that appear, each in the appropriate color.

"Good," says Dr. Rogers, as the next PowerPoint slide is projected. The words appear again, but now in different colors, so that *blue* appears in green type, the word *red* in yellow, and so forth.

"Say the color of the word, but ignore the word," Dr. Rogers reminds them. There is hesitation as participants, still standing on their foam pads, pause for thought. The unison of response is not quite as crisp now.

"Blue . . . no, wait, yellow."

The brainteasers are part of the Stroop Test, a series of drills typically used in laboratory settings to test a person's capacity to direct attention. Incorporating these mental exercises into what is ostensibly a fitness class is based on the idea that so-called cognitive distraction drills can help improve balance.

"You're trying to accomplish two things at once here," explains Dr. Rogers. "That's what we've done. We're distracting the person from focusing on their balance."

And in the process, you're putting greater demands on their neural system, forcing it to attend to two tasks at once, which in turn can help make it more efficient. We are, to refer back to our previous section, pumping up the BDNF.

"This is pretty cutting-edge stuff," says Robert Topp, PhD, a professor of nursing at Marquette University who has researched the effectiveness of various forms of exercise among older adults. Standing strong, he says, goes beyond what is typically used to improve balance. "Mike," he says, referring to Dr. Rogers, "is trying to train people to concentrate on what they're doing as well as retrain their balance. I think he's onto something really important."

So do we—and not only for fall prevention, which is of course a concern for older adults. But the kind of activities that Dr. Rogers has developed—some call it neural-pathway-activation, others refer to it as sensory-motor training or dual-processing activity—represent a potentially new genre of physical training, beyond the usual fitness triad of aerobic exercise, resistance training, and flexibility.

We believe that this kind of neural-physical exercise is very much part of heart-brain health.

Now you might be thinking *What? Another kind of exercise on top of what these guidelines are already recommending? Am I supposed to spend my whole day working out?*

Not at all. The kind of training that challenges your brain and neural system as well as your heart isn't difficult to incorporate into a basic exercise routine. In fact, these movements are kind of fun!

You can get a sense of this kind of training immediately. When you brush your teeth tonight, try standing with one foot in front of the other. Then close your eyes. Requires a little adjusting, right? Feels different, even a bit strange? That's your brain reacting to and then reprogramming to perform an activity in a new and unfamiliar position and with one of its key senses—sight—suddenly unavailable.

How do we incorporate this into your overall program of physical activity? To do that, let us return briefly to the guidelines.

EXERCISE FOR YOUR HEART AND BRAIN: PISCATELLA'S POINTERS ON PUTTING IT ALL TOGETHER

How do you construct an exercise regimen that works for you? Like a lot of fitness and health professionals, I like the formula called FITT.

The *F* stands for *Frequency*. The American College of Sports Medicine says that it takes three days a week of more vigorous exercise to attain cardiovascular fitness. For heart health, I suggest that as your goal (although you need to build up to that goal gradually).

The *I* stands for *Intensity*. How hard are you exercising? If you are walking, for example, it should be more than a casual stroll. One hundred steps a minute is "moderate" intensity, while 130 steps a minute is "vigorous." I also believe that a combination of moderate and high-intensity exercise (HIT) can be beneficial. An example would be to walk five minutes at a moderate pace, then two minutes at a vigorous pace, then back to five minutes at a moderate pace, and so on (breaking up your exercise like that also helps keep you focused and motivated).

I'm not saying you should be doing all-out sprints here—just intense enough exercise that you can feel the effort. (One oft-used cue to gauge ideal aerobic intensity is that it should be easy enough that you can still converse but hard enough that you can't sing.)

By the way, to step back into the research for a moment, one of Dr. Sabbagh's colleagues, Jeff Burns, MD, of the University of Kansas Medical Center (KU) has done some very impressive research on the link between exercise and Alzheimer's, showing how this variable in the fitness formula—intensity—matters. In a 2015 study on the link between exercise and brain function, Dr. Burns and his KU colleagues found that those who exercised with greater intensity had the most improvements in visual-spatial learning, the ability to perceive where objects are in space and their distance from each other, as well as increased attention levels and ability to focus.

The first *T* in the FITT formula stands for *Time*. While we noted earlier that overall health benefits can be derived from very short bouts of activity, the gold standard for achieving the kind of heart-health results we outlined earlier is forty-five minutes.

While a little more aggressive than the Health and Human Services guidelines, that should be your goal. Not at first, though—you don't *start* by trying to exercise nonstop for forty-five minutes. Dr. Sabbagh recommends something closer to the federal guidelines to start out with. He recommends to his patients that they begin with ten to fifteen minutes of brisk walking and gradually build up from there, adding one to two minutes per day each week. "Consistency over strenuousness," he says—and I agree.

The second *T* in the FITT formula stands for *Type.* There are many flavors of exercise out there. We talk about walking and running because they are the most accessible. Of course, you could also ride a bike or take a spin class, swim or row, or participate in an active sport. To build strength, there are many forms of resistance and core training, plus wonderful ways to increase your flexibility, such as yoga (which has other calming and centering benefits as well).

As the old adage says, "the best exercise is the one you'll do!"

YOUR NEW BRAIN-BOOSTING WORKOUT

To this list of familiar types of physical activities, we add a new ingredient: the neural-pathway-activating, balance-type training that, as we have seen from Dr. Rogers' work at Wichita State, can add a one-two punch to the power of your workout, supplementing the brain and heart benefits of physical activity we've discussed in this chapter.

Let's put it all together, starting with the kind of heart-challenging, brain-health-abetting exercise Joe and Dr. Sabbagh have just described. It could be brisk walking; it could be running—or a combination of walking and intervals of jogging.

When you've finished (as noted, beginners should start initially with ten minutes and then gradually build up to forty-five minutes), cool down with a few minutes of easy walking and gentle stretching.

Your muscles are warm, and the blood is flowing—and with it that brain-fertilizing BDNF. Now let's challenge it!

Find a tree, a pole, or a wall for support. Standing erect and with the palm of one hand on the supporting surface, close your eyes and slowly raise your left knee, lifting your leg off the ground. Count slowly to thirty. Then switch legs and repeat.

You've done your first basic balance movement. Your brain is already responding, rewiring circuits to respond.

Now it's simply a question of upping the game a little bit each time. After your next aerobic workout, add fifteen seconds to your one-legged stands, and the time after that, another fifteen seconds, so that you are now standing—with support—for sixty seconds on each leg.

Standing on one leg for an extended period without support sounds easier than it actually is, as you may discover. You might feel like you're suddenly on a rickety foundation. But the brain will adjust, and by your third or fourth session, depending on your age and existing condition, you'll likely be ready to let go of the training wheels.

One more iteration of this basic move: once you can stand unsupported, eyes closed, for sixty seconds on each leg, try turning your head slowly back and forth during each iteration. Don't do it too quickly; you don't want to get dizzy or strain your neck. Just a slow, gradual, side-to-side rotation as you balance on one leg, unsupported.

More challenge for the brain.

But it's a challenge your brain will rise to, perhaps faster than you realize.

"Most people see improvement fairly quickly with these kinds of movements," says Dr. Rogers. "They get more and more confident."

YOUR ADVANCED BRAIN-BOOSTING WORKOUT

This new kind of training is being recognized by fitness professionals. "We call it 'balance training,'" says Bob Phillips, a personal trainer certified by the National Strength and Conditioning Association. "But it's really something more complex."

In the last couple of years, Phillips has begun incorporating this kind of brain-boosting work into the regimens of his one-on-one clients. "It takes them out of their comfort zone," he says. "It forces them to do two things at once, and in the process, it's helping them to become neurally efficient."

Phillips often starts his clients out with basics—like standing on one leg—but, as they progress, he employs an array of props, including wobble boards and the round-on-one-side, flat-on-the-other balls known as BOSUs. Sometimes he'll play catch with a small medicine ball as his client stands on a foam surface, like the participants in Dr. Rogers' class.

But you can do a more advanced brain workout on your own using just a broomstick and a rubber ball. Phillips recommends starting these exercises only after two or three weeks of doing the single-leg stands and the evolutions for it that we just described.

Broomstick Kayaking

After you've finished your aerobic work and cooldown, take your broomstick in both hands at shoulder width, using an overhand grip. Begin to form a figure-eight motion with the broomstick, as if you're kayaking. "You want to visualize it as if you are actually on a kayak," Phillips says. "Try to be rhythmic and smooth." Do this for sixty seconds. Rest a minute, and repeat.

It might take your brain a couple of times to get that fluid motion. But once you're figure-eighting your way along like the kayak version of an air guitar player, challenge yourself by standing on one leg while you do it:

first the right for sixty seconds, then the left for the same amount of time. It's not easy, at least not at first—and of course, that's the point.

Single-Leg Ball Toss

Add this one to the mix after a few sessions of kayaking. You can use a partner for this movement or find a concrete wall that can allow you to rebound a rubber ball. (Try a palm-sized handball or bounce ball that you can find for just a few dollars at any sporting goods store.)

Standing on your right leg, throw the ball to your partner or against the wall and catch it on one bounce—five times, first with your right hand, then five times with your left. Change legs and do the same.

Comfortable? You shouldn't be, at least not at first! "You're forcing a sort of constant adaptation," Phillips says.

The brain must engage in what Dr. Rogers calls "dual processing"—in this case, focusing on catching and throwing the ball while simultaneously adjusting to the instability of standing on one leg.

It may look and feel strange, admittedly. "It's a little out of the box," Phillips says. "But it's kind of like a game, and my clients love it." One reason they do is because, unlike other forms of exercise, you can see improvements in balance and neural training quickly—a tribute to the plasticity of our brains that, in combination with our aerobic exercise, is really helping you attain a new level of heart-brain fitness.

CHAPTER 6

Step 2

---

*Explore the New Borders of
the Mediterranean Diet*

THE MEDITERRANEAN DIET WAS recently voted to be the overall best diet for the tenth year in a row by a panel of twenty-five medical and nutrition professionals reviewing more than forty popular diets for *U.S. News & World Report.*

A plan that prioritizes eating more fruits and veggies with an accent on lean protein and healthy fat, it rated tops in both the heart health and brain health categories as well as the weight loss and diabetes management categories. Further, it received praise for being easy to follow and budget-friendly.

While the common principles of the diet are more or less the same, there is not just one standard Mediterranean diet. The French, Greeks, Italians, and Spanish are all part of the Mediterranean region but take their own unique approach to eating. To complicate matters, some of the popular "internet" diets claim to be the Mediterranean diet but really aren't.

In this chapter, we explore the varying shoreline of the Mediterranean diet as well as some of the diet's new principles, which are less about what foods are eaten and more about *how* the eating is done. In Mediterranean cultures, for example, food is shared; eating is not rushed. Moreover, the base of the new pyramid is now physical activity, underscoring one of the important points of this book—that optimal health is not "just" about modifications in diet or joining a gym; it's a way of life.

Also in this chapter, we'll include some specific tips not found in many nutrition books. For example, new research suggests that elevation of the amino acid homocysteine increases the risk for both coronary artery disease and Alzheimer's disease, and it's reduced by taking folic acid. We'll talk about how to get more of that in your diet as well as the important role of flavonoids—phytonutrients whose important role in both heart and brain health has been confirmed by research published as recently as May 2020.

We will start, however, by taking a broader look not at the Mediterranean diet but at the way people closer to own our shores tend to eat—the American diet and its implications for our health.

THE NOT-SO-GREAT AMERICAN DIET

Many of us want to develop and sustain what are now called *clean eating* habits because we know that our dietary pattern impacts the duration and quality of our life and our health span. Clean eating avoids highly processed and hyperprocessed foods (which usually contain a lot of sugar, fat, salt, and concocted flavorings), emphasizes whole foods, especially plants and plant-based foods, and includes moderate amounts of lean animal protein. This is an overview description of the Mediterranean diet, which is, in our opinion, the best dietary pattern for extending heart and brain health.

Let's begin by examining the other side of clean eating, a diet pattern that penalizes health span—what we call the Standard American Diet (or SAD, an acronym that kind of sums it up). Favorite foods from fried chicken to prime rib, Thanksgiving gravy to Super Bowl snacks, potato chips to Milky Way chocolate bars, strawberry milkshakes to Coca Cola, McDonald's hamburgers to Krispy Kreme doughnuts are just that . . . favorites!

In the United States, where food is plentiful for most people, it embodies pleasure, home, love, tradition, and entertainment. Whatever the occasion, from births to funerals, food is enjoyed and made part of the event. But food can also have an enormous influence on our long-term physical well-being and therefore our health span: eating a balanced diet is one of the smartest things we can do to ward off or manage disease, maximize good health, and extend health span. More than two hundred years ago, the German poet Goethe summed it up perfectly: "You are what you eat." That concept is more clearly understood today in light of the established relationship between nutrition and health.

Unfortunately, the makeup of our modern diet has little to do with our knowledge about its impact on good health. We are eating significant amounts of animal foods, fast foods, highly processed and hyperprocessed convenience foods, and commercially baked goods, all of which make for a diet too rich in saturated and trans fats, added sugars, salt and sodium, and total calories. At the same time, we're not eating enough fruits, vegetables, beans, and whole grains—foods rich in complex carbohydrates, fiber, and antioxidants.

AN UPSIDE-DOWN DIET

Survey data suggest that 40 percent of Americans eat no fruit or vegetables in any given day, while 80 percent eat no whole grains. And the vegetable figure is worse than it seems, as half of those who claim to eat vegetables cite French fries as the *only* vegetable eaten! It is no wonder that we consume less than half of the fiber recommended by USDA.

Experts estimate that if you eat three meals a day, you get at least one-third of your daily calories outside of your home. About two-thirds of us eat fast food twice a week, and snacks provide 25 percent of our calories. And according to the USDA, 16 percent of men and 13 percent of women ages twenty to thirty-nine eat pizza every single day!

Today, most of what Americans eat is highly processed, packaged, and preprepared meals, snacks, and fast foods, all of which are mass-produced by someone else. Most of us are aware of the overreliance on these foods, made by someone else, in our diet. But did you know that there are three different grades of processed foods?

Hyperprocessed foods are industrially formulated mixtures that little resemble their original plant or animal sources. Good examples are hot dogs and margarine. Hyperprocessed foods supply 63 percent of daily calories and are the main source of added sugars, sodium, and saturated fat. *Highly processed* foods such as peanut butter, pasta, and yogurt supply 30 percent of calories. And *unprocessed* or *minimally processed* foods such as fresh produce, beans, and milk unfortunately supply just 7 percent of daily calories.

HEART-ATTACK CITY

Over the past three decades, the increase in portion size of common foods has become a main contributor to overeating and the current obesity epidemic. A study published in the *Journal of the American Medical Association* showed that a homemade hamburger went from 5.7 ounces in 1977 to 8.4 ounces in 1996. And that trend has continued on through today. In the past forty years, U.S. per capita calorie consumption rose from 2,109 calories per day to 2,568 calories per day. That's the equivalent of adding two slices of Domino's pizza to the daily diet of every American.

It is not hard to take in excess calories when cookies are the size of pancakes, muffins are bigger than baseballs, and soft drinks are large enough to drown in. Supersizing is now the standard. Even one of the most beloved cookbooks in American history, *The Joy of Cooking*, has given in to the trend: recipes that used to feed six in this beloved volume (first published in 1931) now feed only four. A main contributor to overeating is an increase in plate size from a 9.5-inch diameter in the 1970s to an 11.5-inch diameter today. Filling these larger plates to capacity and practicing "clean plate club" habits has caused dramatic increases in daily caloric intake for men, women, and children. "Portion distortion" is a main reason the 2003 adult obesity rate of 32 percent has now climbed to almost 40 percent.

Says the late Dr. Mark Hegsted, former director of the federal government's Human Nutrition Center, "The menu we happen to eat today was never planned on the basis of health. It just grew as the result of our affluence, the efficiency of American farmers, the growth of the processed food and fast food industries, the emergence of sophisticated advertising techniques, and the increased pace of modern life. The fact that we consume it today is no indication that it is balanced or desirable." Echoes registered dietitian Megan Ellison, "What we eat today is the result of daily decisions based on impulse, advertising, convenience, economics, status, taste and cravings—on influences other than positive nutrition."

As a result, the Standard American Diet has a huge impact on our health space. It is linked to five of the ten leading causes of death—coronary heart disease, cancer, high blood pressure, stroke, and type 2 diabetes—and the nation's leading ailment, obesity (and as we will see later in this chapter, it has consequences for our brain health as well).

Says former surgeon general, the late C. Everett Koop, "As diseases of nutritional deficiency have diminished, they have been replaced by diseases of dietary excess and imbalance. Americans are gobbling their way to an early grave."

WHY DO WE EAT THIS WAY?

Clearly, most people understand that the contemporary Standard American Diet can be hazardous to health, longevity, and health span. But only 34 percent describe themselves as being "health conscious" in terms of their eating habits. Why, then, do so many of us eat so poorly?

While a number of factors influence food choices, five stand out. The first is the *chronic stress* that is endemic to our hurried and harried modern way of life. Society today is pressure-packed, strung out, out of time, and chronically stressed, often driving us to choose processed and fast foods on the spur of the moment and without thought to health. Says Evelyn Tribole, RD, "Stressed out people often eat on the run and settle for what is available quickly, from restaurants, take-outs, and food stores. Health and nutrition are not factors they consider." Research also shows that chronic stress can influence eating habits. Experts say that people who reach for food in response to stress do so as a means of self-medication. "It's nature's way of getting you to feel better," says Dr. Judith Wurtman at McLean Hospital. "Food often acts as an edible tranquillizer."

The second major influence is a *toxic environment*. We are surrounded by a limitless supply of tasty, inexpensive, high-calorie food, usually sold and served in oversized portions. "Unhealthy choices are available on every corner, from fast-food restaurants to shopping malls and movie theaters, and it compounds the problem of how to eat healthy," according to Dr. Kelly Brownell, a leading obesity expert at Duke University. "Modern society is a toxic environment for making healthy food choices," he states. "Everywhere you turn there is an opportunity to eat poorly, backed up by an advertising industry that encourages overeating."

A third influence is a *smorgasbord approach to health information*. There always seem to be opposing facets to the science of healthy eating. Shrimp were once "out"; now they are "in," for example. Americans tend to pick and choose what science to believe and recommendations to practice based on what we want to hear. The call to eat less fat (which was actually a call to eat less *saturated* fat), if implemented properly (less red meat, more fruits and vegetables), could have led us to a healthier society. Instead, it led us to SnackWell's and other low-fat, high-calorie junk foods manufactured by the food industry to give us what we wanted. As long as the label said "low fat," it met our self-selected criterion for good health. And of course, because of the high level of added sugars in these foods, it met our sweet-tooth desires.

An unintended result of the pick-and-choose method of evaluating dietary science was to move us from one problem (heart disease promoted by a diet rich in saturated fats) to two new problems (obesity and type 2 diabetes promoted by refined carbohydrate foods rich in added sugars.) In fact, it could be argued that Americans are sicker than ever. Consider this:

- Eighty-six million people are now prediabetic. (90 percent do not even know that they are in this category.)
- Almost 70 percent of the population is overweight or obese.
- About 54 percent of adults have abdominal obesity.

Fourth are the *economic and biological forces* that have led to a growth in fast food consumption. The economics are easy to understand: fast food is cheap and plentiful. But biology also plays a role. We are biologically predisposed from prehistoric times to consume a diet high in calories, sugar, and fat—just what is found in a Happy Meal and other fast foods. Says Dr. Marion Nestle at New York University, "When you eat a Big Mac, your blood sugar soars. Your brain then releases a flood of chemicals, such as dopamine, that induce pleasure and contribute to a tendency to eat compulsively. This can produce cravings for foods rich in salt, fat and sugar that can be addictive."

And finally, a critical factor is that much of America has *stopped cooking at home*. This may have been temporarily halted by the pandemic, when we had no choice but to eat at home. But at this writing, my bet is that when one spouse says to another in an old joke, "What are you making for dinner?" the response is "Reservations!" Because of longer average work hours and more two-worker households, we often find our schedules maxed out, with less time left for home-cooked meals. Eating competes with many other activities in our fragmented lives. As a result, many people are no longer inclined to shop, cook, or make food choices based on good nutrition. They often eat on the run and settle for what is available quickly, from eat-in and takeout restaurants, packaged and ready-to-eat foods, and grocery stores. Data show that at 4 p.m. on any given day, 70 percent of Americans do not know what they are having for dinner that night. The bottom line is that many have simply traded nutrition for convenience. Where are the fresh fruits and vegetables? Where are the whole grains, legumes, and other healthy foods in this scenario? Not in the American kitchen or on the American dinner table.

"The tragedy in this situation," says columnist Mark Bittman, "is that there is a simple solution: cook more at home." Healthy eating means making a commitment to cook more meals at home. And that is not too difficult to do. Indeed, there are many recipes that are simple and easy to prepare. How we eat—whether we cook at home or grab fast-food takeout—matters as much as what we eat. Does that mean preparing twenty-one meals a week in your own kitchen? No, of course not. But it does mean cooking most meals yourself. Sure, everyone today is time-pressed, but if good health and extended health span are priorities, you have to find time to cook.

DEVELOP A HEALTHY PERSPECTIVE: THINK "HABITS," NOT "DIETS"

"Ready, fire, aim" is not a good plan for making any healthy lifestyle change, especially when it comes to what you will eat on a day-by-day basis. The opportunity to improve your habits and to achieve successful aging increases if you first prepare for making those changes.

Eating healthier, exercising regularly, and consciously managing your stress do not happen automatically. That's why preparation is so important. From the standpoint of healthy eating, here are a few basic things to consider during the planning stage before taking any action:

First of all, let's think less about "diets" and more about "habits." The word *diet* has a singular connotation. It's a short-term weight reduction program, a means of shedding pounds by restricting calories eaten. The formula that most often moves a diet book to a *New York Times* best-seller list is the promise of some new, grand epiphany regarding a scapegoat ("Never eat this food!"), a silver bullet ("Always eat this food!"), or both. The author has managed to figure out what the rest of us missed: how to achieve effortless success. Of course, if this were true, there would be no need for new diet books. The answers would be in the thousands of diet books already published. As one doctor told me, "We are smart enough to put a man on the moon, but when it comes to diet books, we're dumb as sticks."

People who want to lose weight quickly (often magically) periodically go "on" then "off" a fad diet until either the "on" or—more likely—the "off" eventually wins. Comedian Sandra Bergeson, in her *I Hate to Diet Dictionary*, defines *fad dieting* as "the all-consuming obsession with the food you shouldn't have eaten yesterday, but did; the food you have eaten today, but shouldn't have; and the food you shouldn't eat tomorrow, but probably will."

When we refer to "diet," I do not mean the typical fad diet. I'm actually talking about a "diet pattern," a much broader way to look at how we eat (as reflected in the latest dietary guidelines). Healthy eating is not an isolated event. Instead, it is part of a healthy cascade of habits including regular exercise, managed stress, better sleep, more energy, and, yes, better food decisions. It is not a magical diet formula constructed by the fad diet industry that focuses on individual elements and requires much willpower for success.

Fad dieting can create major problems. We are often so obsessed about what we are eating immediately on our "diet" that we fail to recognize reality. In the world of advertising fantasies, you can change the way you eat for a week or two and be thin for a lifetime. In the real world, this concept is a sham.

There are many good reasons not to diet even if weight is lost in the short term. One is that fad diets can place you in a catch-22 situation. If you come off the diet, you regain the weight. If you stay on the diet, it can have a negative impact on health. Few fad diets have been tested in studies.

The most obvious reason to avoid fad dieting is that it doesn't work. Research shows that while weight (much of it body fluids rather than body fat) may be lost in the short term, few dieters keep the weight off in the long term. One study of "high protein, low carbohydrate" diets suggests that 94 percent of participants not only regained their lost weight after one year; they put on a few extra pounds. This has been the experience of my friend, Dave. He initially lost forty pounds on the Atkins diet but a year later had gained eighty pounds. Fad diets don't work.

Over the past sixty years or so, thousands of quick weight-loss fad diets have been promoted. (Remember the grapefruit and cigarette diet?) If any one of them had been effective—if the cabbage soup diet had worked!—we would be a nation of skinny folks. But we are not. Instead, we are at the top of the list of the fattest countries on earth. Why? Because fad diets don't work.

Dr. David Katz of Yale University's Prevention Research Center has become a searing critic of popular fad diets: "The empty promises of diet crazes are more than annoying and confusing; they are dangerous. I really at times feel like crying, when I think that we're paying for ignorance with human lives. At times, I hate the people who are promising the moon and the stars with certainty. I hate knowing that the next person is already rubbing his or her hands together with the next fad to make it on the bestseller list."

The bottom line is that there is little relationship between fad dieting and good health. You don't need a "diet" to extend health span; you need a healthy "diet pattern," a long-term manner of eating that will produce positive results. Anyone can change the way she eats for a week. The real goal is to improve your eating habits for a lifetime.

SOUND NUTRITIONAL SCIENCE
AND COMMON SENSE

I'm sure that you've heard much of this before. How could you not? There has never been a time where there has been more information available on healthy eating—from best-selling diet books to infomercials for cleanses and secret tips in glossy magazines. Unfortunately, most are not based on credible nutritional science. When watching medical experts tout the addition or subtraction of one nutrient as deliverance—only to change the channel and hear someone equally thoroughly credentialed touting the opposite—it can be tempting to write off nutrition advice altogether. This month, we hear something is good, and the next, we almost expect to hear it's bad. Why not assume the latest research will all eventually be nullified and just close our eyes and eat whatever tastes best?

It is important, then, to base your dietary decisions on science from reliable sources such as the American Heart Association, the Academy of Nutrition and Dietetics, and the National Cancer Institute. I particularly like newsletters such as *Nutrition Action, the Berkeley Wellness Letter* and the *Tufts Newsletter*. Be aware that some studies are funded by food manufacturers and that some authors take a "man bites dog" approach, presenting contrarian information as a marketing "hook."

JOE'S JOURNEY: DEVELOPING A
TASTE FOR GOOD HEALTH

The longest and most challenging part of my journey from heart patient to heart-health advocate began in the days immediately following my bypass surgery in 1977.

As I returned to my family to recuperate, the reality of our situation hit home. I knew that the first big step in my road back was to change my diet, but how? And as part of a family of four, I realized that I couldn't expect to be following one way of eating while Bernie and the kids ate differently. How were we going to eat? Was there a diet that would both satisfy the family and boost cardiac health?

We tried to design something on our own and failed. The problem was the taste (or lack thereof) in many so-called healthy foods. I remember the first lunch Bernie and I shared after returning home: a dry turkey sandwich, no mayonnaise, on cardboard-like bread. "I may have survived surgery," I told Bernie, "but I don't think I'll survive lunch!" That taught us a basic premise: if the healthy food isn't appealing and doesn't taste great, no one will eat it, not even a heart patient.

It was then that we decided to investigate two of the most popular diet concepts: low-fat and low-carbohydrate (high-fat) diets.

We first considered extremely low-fat diets, many of which contained less than 10 percent of calories from fat. This diet pattern seemed reasonable to me, as many experts linked low-fat eating to improved heart health. Much of that thinking came as a result of a 1977 U.S. Senate committee's landmark recommendations—*Dietary Goals for the United States.* One of the primary directives, based on the latest information at that time, was to cut fat consumption to reduce heart-attack risk. (This perspective has since been debunked.) With nearly one million heart-attack deaths each year, it was clear that we had to do something. The goal of reducing fat was codified in 1980, when the USDA issued its first dietary guidelines and the American Heart Association and others took up the mantra.

At that time, it seemed imperative for me as a heart patient to follow those recommendations and consume an extremely low-fat diet. So instituting a dietary pattern with less than 10 percent of calories from fat became a goal of mine. However, after a period of time, I was faced with two problems. The first is that I began to question the efficacy of extremely low-fat eating. The fact is that reducing or eliminating fat from my diet didn't feel right. How was it that Italians, Spanish, French, Greek, and other Mediterranean peoples could eat as they did—a diet routinely about 40 percent fat or more—yet still have low levels of heart disease?

In addition, such diets were often extremely restrictive, usually banning favorite, forbidden foods forever. Often this advice doesn't produce the result that we desire. Here is an example. A few months after bypass surgery, I had a checkup with a dietitian who was a low-fat guru. When I asked her about eating a healthy diet, she gave me two sheets of paper. The green-colored sheet (green for "go") listed all the foods I should eat—fruits, vegetables, whole grains . . . you know the list. The red-colored sheet (red for "stop") provided me with a list of banned foods, many of which were favorites—chocolate, cheese, hot dogs, and pizza. Then to top it off, for she knew me well, she said, "And don't have another Oreo cookie for the rest of your life!"

The result was that she highlighted and identified a food that I would now kill for. Or as Evelyn Tribole, RD, puts it, "The Food Police bring out the Diet Rebel." I held out for two or three days, but Oreo cookies were constantly on my mind. Then on the fourth day, I found myself eating my way through an entire package. At that point, I was ready to give up on any attempt to eat a healthy diet, as I knew that forbidden foods would creep in. "What was the point of even trying?" I asked. (This is the "what the heck" factor. I may as well eat the whole package since I already broke the rules.)

What I learned from this experience was that there were few, if any, absolutes. The fact is that had I learned how to fit an Oreo or two into my low-fat diet, I would have done a better job at maintaining a healthy dietary pattern. That is where the concept of balance takes place. A healthy dietary pattern provides such a balance and allows for indulgences. That's important when you are eating for a lifetime.

After an unproductive experience with low-fat diets, I gravitated toward "high-protein, low-carbohydrate" diets as proposed by best-selling author Dr. Robert Atkins and others. ("High protein" actually translates to "high fat.") The diet surely sounded tasty—bacon, cheeseburgers, and protein shakes—and a number of my friends had lost weight on this regimen. But two things caused me to dismiss this high-fat dietary pattern. First, many of those friends who had lost weight on such diets put the weight back on (and then some) when they came off the diet. So "low-carb, high-fat" eating was not a permanent lifestyle change. Next, I became concerned about the elevated saturated fat content of red meat, whole-milk dairy products, and other such foods central to this way of eating. I was aware that a host of studies suggest less inflammation and heart disease resulted when saturated fat is reduced and replaced by unsaturated fat. As regarding health span, numerous studies show that the longest-lived, most vital populations vary widely in total fat consumption, but none have a high intake of saturated fat. It made no sense, therefore, for me as a heart patient to consume that much saturated fat. There was no reason to eat in a way that would cause my cholesterol to soar and my cardiac risk to increase. I abandoned it.

I felt good about not subscribing to extremely low-fat or high-fat diets, but Bernie and I still did not have a solution. It was obvious that we were struggling with what to eat, and once again Bernie's sound thinking rescued us: "Let's take a break from trying to force new dietary habits on our life and use the time to determine (1) which diets pattern gives us the best cardiac protection and (2) how to translate that information into practical, daily meals." I agreed.

It was time for some sound medical advice, so I visited with my cardiologist. While many doctors are not well-versed in nutrition, my cardiologist was. He got straight to the point: "Joe, you should look at the Mediterranean diet, characterized by the traditional cooking style of countries bordering the Mediterranean Sea. Unlike other diets based on food rules or absolutes (no fat, no carbs, etc.), the Mediterranean diet is not a 'diet.' Instead, it is a healthy eating pattern based on moderation and balance." According to the current dietary guidelines, "It provides an adaptable framework in which individuals can enjoy foods that meet their personal, cultural and traditional preferences." Its underlying principle is that good food and good health go together.

I found that the Mediterranean diet is not simply about eating; it is more about a lifestyle that also recognizes the importance of being physically active and enjoying meals with family and friends. I like the fact that it establishes a way of eating within a way of life that fosters good health. "We shouldn't be thinking about individual foods in isolation," says Dr. Alice Lichtenstein of Tufts University.

"We need to help people put together a healthy dietary pattern, looking at the whole picture at once." The Mediterranean diet does just that.

My doctor was also impressed with the science behind the Mediterranean diet and the connection to better health, citing its robust scientific connection to good long-term heart and brain health, and the extent to which it dramatically decreases the risk of chronic disease. In addition, it is clearly associated with significant lengthening of health span and longevity.

In the next section of this chapter, we will cite some of the many studies that have shown the value of the Mediterranean diet for the brain as well as the heart.

Suffice it to say, the evidence is robust—which is why the USDA's *Dietary Guidelines for Americans* now recommends the Mediterranean diet as an eating pattern that can help promote health and health span and prevent disease.

Once I had credible science, it was time to apply common sense to my actions. My default position from early on was a middle-of-the-road, moderate, and balanced dietary pattern based very much on the global principles of a Mediterranean-style diet: focus not on one thing but on the whole diet. Be aware of the impact of nutrients on health, but center your dietary pattern on foods. I have been consistent with this in my personal life and in my books. My eating pattern has incorporated a variety of foods: fruits, vegetables, beans, nuts, fish, olive oil, lean protein, whole grains, berries, dairy products, and even wine. I have centered my selections on fresh, local, and in-season whole foods and reduced or eliminated refined, processed, packaged, and ready-to-eat foods, particularly those containing numerous additives, unhealthy trans fat, and added sugar. I have eaten well with "real food." My cardiologist once remarked, "Joe, you have been eating and recommending the Mediterranean diet since before it was called the Mediterranean diet."

In addition, the litmus test for many of my dietary decisions was "what works" for me, what foods tasted great, were easy to prepare, and resulted in good cholesterol; blood pressure; and weight numbers. In other words, foods that would allow me to stick with healthy eating long-term. Bernie and I were well aware of the principles of the Mediterranean diet, as we lived as students in Rome and ate such a diet. It worked great in Italy, but it would need some modification if it were to translate successfully to the United States.

For example, the Mediterranean diet included meat about once a month, fish and chicken once a week or so, and milk virtually never. But I liked meat and milk! If I had to restrict meat to once a month and give up milk altogether, the diet was doomed to fail. But science showed that you didn't have to be "100 percent in" to reap health benefits. So instead of adopting the Mediterranean diet as it was traditionally eaten, we adapted it to our way of life and food preferences. It became a *Mediterranean-style* diet that took the principles of healthy Mediterranean eating and applied them to the American lifestyle. For example, I ate meat, fish, and poultry more often than Mediterranean people do but a lot less frequently than the typical American. And I ate more fruit, vegetables, beans, and whole grains than the typical American. (Fat-free milk was also included in my new diet.)

This approach to healthy eating worked for me. First and foremost, it satisfied my need for food that tasted great and that I wanted to eat. I didn't feel short-changed. The reality is that there are no magic foods or quick-fix solutions for eating healthy. Foods are not inherently totally "good" or "bad," as in you should always eat or you never should eat. Some, however, are better choices than others (such as olive oil rather than stick margarine.) My belief is that all food is good food. It's just that some foods are eaten in unhealthy amounts.

Next, it supported my cardiac health. I never lost sight of the fact that the risk of death from heart disease could decrease by 30 percent by eating this diet. Indeed, I believe I would not have made it to forty-four years post bypass surgery if I had eaten in any other way. As mentioned earlier, the Mediterranean diet was voted overall best diet for the tenth year in a row—you can add my vote (and that of Bernie's and my cardiologist's) to that as well.

DR. SABBAGH: THE SCIENCE BEHIND THE MEDITERRANEAN DIET'S HEART AND BRAIN BENEFITS

While it is not the only diet that can promote heart and brain health, the Mediterranean diet is the one I generally recommend. Why? I'm a researcher as well as a clinician, so I want evidence. And there is plenty to back this eating plan. Here are just a few of the summaries of important studies that have demonstrated the diet's efficacy in every aspect of health but particularly on the brain and the heart and what Joe referred to earlier as health span—one's quality of life.

Research on women published in the *Annals of Internal Medicine* found that those who followed the Mediterranean diet lived longer and with an extended health span. The diets of over ten thousand women in their late fifties and early sixties were examined and recorded in this study. At the end of a fifteen-year follow-up, the study showed that those who followed the Mediterranean diet had a 40 percent better chance of living past age seventy compared with those who did not follow the Mediterranean diet.

These so-called healthy agers were also found to be free from eleven chronic diseases, including heart disease, kidney failure, cancer, type 2 diabetes, Alzheimer's disease, and Parkinson's disease. Furthermore, they showed no physical disabilities, no signs of cognitive impairment, and no signs of mental health problems.

The Mediterranean diet works particularly well with older adults. One of the definitive studies on the Mediterranean diet was conducted by Dr. Ramon Estruch at the University of Barcelona on 7,500 people, mostly in their sixties and seventies. All participants were at risk for developing heart disease. Most were overweight, and many had diabetes, high blood pressure, elevated cholesterol, and other risk factors. Participants were divided into three groups. The first group ate the Mediterranean diet and also ate an extra ounce of mixed nuts (walnuts, hazelnuts, and almonds) every day. The second group followed the Mediterranean diet and also ate five daily tablespoons of extra-virgin olive oil (one of my favorites). The third group followed a lower-fat diet than the two other groups.

The magnitude of the diet's benefits startled experts. It found that *about 30 percent of strokes and death from heart disease could be prevented in high-risk people by eating the Mediterranean diet.* (That, by the way, is more protection than that conferred by statin drugs!) Researchers were impressed with the study because it used meaningful endpoints. "It did not simply look at risk factors like cholesterol or hypertension or weight," says Dr. Rachel Johnson of the University of Vermont. "It looked at heart attacks and strokes and death. At the end of the day, that is what really matters." Dr. Steven Nissen, chairman of the department of cardiovascular medicine at the Cleveland Clinic Foundation, finds this data to be encouraging to patients in light of the sometimes conflicting information on the healthiest way to eat. "Now along comes this group," he says, "and does a gigantic study in Spain that says you can eat a nicely balanced diet with fruits and vegetable and olive oil and lower heart disease by 30 percent. And you can actually enjoy life. That is great news."

It is indeed. As are the findings of research from colleagues in my discipline of neurology. Work by Columbia University's Nikolaos Scarmeas and colleagues has shown the value of this approach to eating for brain health. One of Dr. Scarmeas's studies followed more than 2,200 people without dementia for up to thirteen years, with an average tracking time of four years. They gave each participant a Mediterranean diet score ranging from zero to nine. Beyond slowing the development of Alzheimer's, adherence to the Mediterranean diet seemed to provide a link to a slower rate of cognitive decline, even after adjustments for other variables.

Writing three years later in the *Journal of the American Medical Association*, Dr. Scarmeas reported on further research, showing that adherence to the Mediterranean diet is associated with a reduction in the risk of mild cognitive impairment (MCI)—defined by the Mayo Clinic as a transitional stage between the cognitive decline of normal aging and the more serious memory problems caused by dementia or Alzheimer's disease—and, perhaps more significantly, in the reduction of risk of conversion of MCI to Alzheimer's disease.

That study also found that the higher the adherence to the Mediterranean diet, the lower the risk for Alzheimer's, with the top one-third of subjects who continued to follow the diet having a 68 percent lower risk of developing Alzheimer's, compared with the bottom third who went off it.

What's particularly striking to me is that these effects were seen even when taking into account other variables such as age, gender, ethnicity, education, caloric intake, BMI, and ApoE genotype.

Why is this? What about the Mediterranean diet makes it so beneficial? The short answer is that we're not exactly sure, but some speculate that simply making the healthy food choices that are a part of this diet may improve cholesterol and blood sugar levels and overall blood vessel health, which may, in turn, reduce the risk of MCI or Alzheimer's disease. This line of thought speaks directly to the premise of this book—that brain and heart health are deeply related.

Whatever the reason, the applause for the Mediterranean diet is deservedly long and sustained. But we should again point out that it's not the only one that can be effective: research suggests the whole-food, plant-based diet (WFPB) is beneficial for the body and brain. Then there's the ketogenic diet, which is controversial but has shown to help reduce symptoms of dementia and is likely best suited for the dementia state.

Here's a little more information on these diets, both of which may have benefits:

The *whole-food plant-based diet (WFPB)* is filled with whole foods (unprocessed, unrefined, high fiber, low sugar) and plants (green, leafy vegetables). The concept of "whole" foods is this: eat plant-based foods in forms that are as close to their natural state as possible. Restaurants and other foodies like to call this farm-to-table food. In other words, the closer the source of the food you consume and the less it is altered by chemicals and additives, the healthier it is for your body. Eat a variety of vegetables, fruits, raw nuts, seeds, beans, and legumes and avoid salt, vegetable oil, and sugar. The aim is to get 80 percent of your calories from carbohydrates, 10 percent from fats, and 10 percent from protein. That's the WFPB shortlist. WFPB diets have been shown to robustly reduce cardiovascular disease. Studies are currently underway to determine if they help reduce Alzheimer's disease.

While some might think of it as the trendy diet of the moment, *ketogenic diets* have actually been around for decades. In fact, prescribing the ketogenic diet is a standard treatment for certain forms of epilepsy. Thus the ketogenic diet is not new to neurology, just new to Alzheimer's disease. The logic for this comes from the premise that Alzheimer's might be a form of "type 3 diabetes," with insulin resistance occurring exclusively in the brain. By adhering to a ketogenic diet, proponents say, there might be an improvement in brain metabolic function because the energy source for nutrition would not rely on insulin.

The "keto" diet is a high-fat, low-carb diet in which the body produces ketones in the liver that are used as energy. The thinking is that by lowering the intake of carbs, the body is induced into a state known as "ketosis"—a natural process the body initiates to help us survive when food intake is low. During this state, we produce ketones, which are produced from the breakdown of fats in the liver. By overloading the body with fats and taking away carbohydrates, the body will burn ketones as the primary energy source. Optimal ketone levels are said to improve health, promote weight loss, and have physical and mental performance benefits.

In short, the ketogenic diet provides alternative fuel for the brain. But alternative fuel may only be effective at certain stages of Alzheimer's disease, so it remains to be seen if this diet should be used if there is no cognitive impairment. Currently, we do not know what impact the ketogenic diet has during various stages, from MCI to Alzheimer's disease, but I think it makes more sense *for* people with symptomatic dementia, not as protection against it.

Also, it is quite difficult to adhere to the keto diet for long periods of time, whereas the Mediterranean and WFPB diets are easier to maintain.

Thus I prefer the Mediterranean—and its variants, the Dietary Approaches to Stop Hypertension (DASH) and Mediterranean-DASH Intervention for Neurodegenerative Delay (MIND)—as well as the WFPB diets for optimal heart-brain health. One study, reported by the Mayo Clinic, examined whether following a Mediterranean diet, the DASH diet designed to treat high blood pressure, or the MIND diet, which combined aspects of both, could reduce the risk of Alzheimer's disease. The results showed that people who strictly followed *any* of the three diets had a lower risk of Alzheimer's disease. Moreover, even modest adoption of the MIND diet approach, such as eating two vegetable servings a day, two berry servings a week, and one fish meal a week, appeared to lower the risk of Alzheimer's disease.

Those findings are a good reminder that, as with the "small steps" approach to physical activity that we discussed in the last chapter, the same holds true for nutrition: even making a few adjustments to your diet is a good start—especially with a diet like this. Unlike some eating plans, the Mediterranean diet is sustainable. It is that rare diet that doesn't make you feel like you're being deprived of something you like. On this diet, you are eating delicious, fresh, and satisfying foods and getting huge health benefits. That's the proverbial win-win.

Before we turn to some specific tasty and heart/brain-healthy eating tips, here are my overall suggestions. And yes, these are also core recommendations of the Mediterranean diet. Follow these guidelines and you'll be getting a benefit to both your heart and your brain:

Reduce saturated fat. Saturated fat has been implicated in both Alzheimer's and coronary artery disease.

In other words, it's bad for your heart *and* it's bad for your brain. Reduce these saturated fats by reducing your consumption of red meat, butter, fried foods, and lard.

Increase fatty fish consumption. We just suggested cutting down on the saturated "bad" fats in your diet by reducing red meat. What do you replace that with? I suggest salmon, sardines, tuna, anchovies, mackerel, and herring. All are rich in omega-3 fatty acids—the "good" fats. Increasing your intake of these fish—popular in many Mediterranean cultures, by the way—can have big cardiovascular and cognitive benefits.

Increase olive oil consumption. Olive oil is a monounsaturated fat and is a key component of the Mediterranean diet. I'm a big fan of it—and I tell all my patients to increase their consumption. Again, as with so much of this diet, it's an easy recommendation to make because olive oil is such a delicious addition to any dish.

Tips for Tasty, Healthy Eating, Mediterranean-Style

Here are some further tips on adopting the Mediterranean diet from nutritionist Tracy Stopler, MS, RD, who teaches in the Health and Sports Sciences Department at New York's Adelphi University.

Spices and Herbs Are Your Friends

With highly processed foods being eliminated, some may find the Mediterranean diet a tad plain at first. Fresh herbs, dried herbs, and spices all add an extra element of flavor to a dish. Don't be afraid to use them, just as those who have followed this way of eating for centuries have used them to spice up their meals.

Nuts and Veggies Are a Perfect Snack

Carrots, peppers, cucumbers, olives, walnuts, almonds, and Brazil nuts are all nutrient-dense options. The vegetables provide a satisfying crunch along with sufficient dietary fiber. They can be eaten alone or paired with hummus, tahini, or yogurt dip. The nuts are a simple, satiating option. Both are accessible, nutritious snacks that are also easy to travel with.

Don't Be Afraid to Eat Out

Eating out and taking out food can seem intimidating—even when there's not a pandemic! Here are a few quick tips to keep in mind when you begin to return to dining out of the home:

- Fish is a great choice. Pair with a baked potato, sweet potato, or whole grain such as brown rice or quinoa. Add vegetables on the side such as broccoli, spinach, or even a side salad.
- Go for the roasted/baked/grilled options.
- Always request olive oil on the side instead of butter, especially if there is a whole grain bread option. If oil is necessary to cook your food, request olive oil.
- Make use of side dishes.

- Vegetables are a large portion of what makes up the Mediterranean diet. If you're stuck somewhere with limited options, use the side dishes offered. Use them to bulk up a salad or make a meal out of them. Roasted carrots, potatoes, or broccoli and sautéed spinach are common side dishes across the board. Ask for a side of rice, grilled chicken, shrimp, or baked salmon and you have yourself a puzzle of a meal.
- Sushi and sashimi are a perfect option. Request to swap out the white rice with brown rice and steer away from any tempura.

Go Easy on the Beans, Lentils, and Legumes at First If You're Not Used to Them

Beans and other legumes are a staple of the Mediterranean diet, says Stopler. If your previous eating habits didn't include frequent amounts of beans or other legumes, you may experience some discomfort. These foods are packed with fiber and protein and are very nutritious. However, people often complain of gas and/or bloating after consuming beans/lentils/legumes. Because of this, many become discouraged and fall off the diet. Start slow. See what you can tolerate and work from there.

There are a few things you can do to make beans more digestible:

- Rinse and soak dry beans/lentils/legumes overnight and rinse them again well before cooking them.

- Cook your beans/lentils/legumes with a piece of kombu. Kombu is a sea vegetable similar to seaweed. It contains enzymes that help break down the components of beans/lentils/legumes that our bodies have a hard time digesting, which leads to bloating/gas/discomfort.
- Protein-rich foods contain the amino acid methionine that converts to homocysteine. Excess levels of homocysteine damage the lining of arteries. Scarred arteries increase cholesterol buildup and can lead to fatal blockages. Vitamins B_6, B_{12}, and folic acid safeguard against elevated serum homocysteine levels by degrading them.
  - *Vitamin B_6* is found in green, leafy vegetables; fish; poultry; nuts; and whole-grain cereals.
  - *Vitamin B_{12}* is found in meat, fish, poultry, eggs, and dairy products (anything that swims, walks, or flies).
  - *Folic acid* is found in green, leafy vegetables; fruits; orange juice; wheat germ; dried beans; and peas.

Tracy has put together a comprehensive selection of meal suggestions and a nutritional analysis that we have included in the back of this book. We urge you to review her delicious suggestions to help make the Mediterranean diet *your* diet.

CHAPTER 7

Step 3

Restful Sleep for Body and Brain

A 2018 ARTICLE IN THE *American Journal of Respiratory and Critical Care Medicine* ticked off the adverse effects of poor sleep: "Insufficient or poor-quality sleep," wrote the study's authors, "affects the immune system, weight management, glucose metabolism, cardiovascular and cerebrovascular health, cognition, work productivity, psychological well-being, and public safety."

Given the breadth of that list of adverse outcomes, one is left wondering if there is any aspect of health *not* impacted by lack of sleep.

"We know what the outcomes are from not having enough sleep," says Dr. Penny Stern, MD, MPH, a lifestyle medicine specialist at Northwell Health in New York. "It's very clear that sleep deficits are linked to many, many problems."

And yet quality and quantity of sleep often seem an afterthought—the last thing on the list of recommended, healthy behaviors.

Growing evidence suggests otherwise, which is why we have included this chapter about sleep right behind exercise and diet in our recommended behaviors for heart and brain health. Not because the other interventions that we discuss in subsequent chapters—stress reduction, cognitive stimulation, and so on—are any less important, but simply because sleep (to use a cultural reference from the seventies and eighties) is like the Rodney Dangerfield of lifestyle: it doesn't get much respect.

In fact, until recently, it used to be almost the opposite. Eight hours in bed was seen as a waste of time by high achievers, who could better use that time to be productive (or so they thought). Lack of sleep used to be a badge of honor, a way to show off how important and busy you were. We now understand such a boast comes at a huge cost to the neuro-cardio system.

At least one hundred million Americans struggle with sleep issues. Lack of shut-eye causes glitches in glucose metabolism and blood pressure and robs neurons of their ability to operate properly. And a sleep-related condition, obstructive sleep apnea, has a hugely significant impact on heart health.

The issue of sleep has been exacerbated by the pandemic. "Insomnia was a problem before COVID-19," said Angela Drake, a UC Davis Health clinical professor in the Department of Psychiatry and Behavioral Sciences. "Now, from what we know anecdotally, the increase is enormous." A June 2020 study in the journal *Sleep Medicine* found that the coronavirus was causing what some call a "second pandemic" of insomnia and sleep issues. The study, conducted in China early in the pandemic by researchers from the Quebec Mental Health University Institute, revealed high rates of clinically significant insomnia, acute stress, anxiety, and depression.

The emergence of what some have called "coronasomnia" underscores the importance of making sleep a higher priority in your plan for optimal brain health.

It was a lesson that coauthor Joe Piscatella learned long before anyone had ever heard of the coronavirus or COVID-19.

JOE'S JOURNEY: ADDING SLEEP TO THE EQUATION

Starting shortly after my coronary bypass surgery in 1977, I began focusing on how to build a heart-healthy lifestyle. The prognosis after the surgery wasn't good, but I wasn't buying it. My family history, my DNA, may have indicated cardiac risk, but I knew (hoped) that living a healthy lifestyle could provide protection.

My focus immediately fell on the big three: diet, exercise, and stress. For about fifteen years, this was my main and only concern: How to eat a healthy, Mediterranean-style diet. How to exercise regularly. How to manage my chronic stress.

As diet, exercise, and stress fell into place, I began to understand that there were other factors—some the result of lifestyle, some not—that could influence cardiac health. A good example is chronic anger. A recent study found that an episode of severe anger was associated with a significantly higher risk of heart attack in the following two hours. Getting so angry that your "blood boils," it seems, may stress your heart and cause your arteries to clog too.

The number of new factors influencing cardiac risk was surprising, none more than insufficient sleep, or insomnia. I had always considered it as primarily a social issue or inconvenience rather than a medical condition that can affect health and well-being. How could sleep be an important factor? That was my thinking because lack of sleep was never a problem for me. Since the surgery, I tended to "sleep like a log." (In retrospect, it might have come about because of my increased exercise, healthier diet, and mind relaxation.) But for many others, it was a significant cardiac risk factor. That's because sleep provides time for the body to restore and recharge. During sleep, blood pressure drops, your heart rate slows, and breathing stabilizes, reducing stress on the heart and allowing it to recover from strain. For the cardiovascular system, insufficient or fragmented sleep, producing a lack of oxygenation, is linked to a host of cardiovascular risks, including, according to the American Heart Association, high blood pressure, diabetes, obesity, and coronary heart disease. Says Dr. Susan Redline of the Harvard Medical School, "Sleep-deprived people have higher blood levels of stress hormones and substances that indicate inflammation, a key player in cardiovascular disease."

The bottom line is that without enough sleep, your risk for heart disease and heart attack goes up—no matter what your age, your weight, or how much you exercise or smoke. At the same time, people who already have high blood pressure, coronary artery disease, heart failure, or a history of stroke tend to sleep more poorly. You just read the staggering statistics on heart health for those who have obstructive sleep especially due to sleep apnea—a condition in which an airway temporarily collapses repeatedly during sleep, depriving the body of oxygen.

More about sleep apnea in a moment. First, let's look at some of the ways that lack of sleep can affect your heart.

HOW LACK OF SLEEP AFFECTS HEART HEALTH

High Blood Pressure

High blood pressure, a prime risk factor for cardiovascular disease, can sometimes be traced to insomnia, particularly difficulty falling or staying asleep. Insomnia affects up to a third of people at some point in their lives.

Blood pressure doesn't always stay constant. A stressful event may cause it to increase; listening to music may cause it to decrease. During normal, healthy sleep, blood pressure drops some 10 to 15 percent, a condition identified as "nocturnal dipping." This allows the body to recover from the stresses of the day, and research highlights its role in cardiovascular health. But insomnia, whether from a lack of sleep or from sleep disruptions, is associated with nondipping, meaning that a person's blood pressure doesn't go down at night. Studies have found that elevated nighttime blood pressure often results in high blood pressure.

Elevated nocturnal blood pressure has been found to be even more predictive of heart problems than high blood pressure during the day. Nondipping has been tied to an increased risk of stroke and heart attack. It's also been linked to kidney problems and reduced blood flow to the brain. In addition, some people with insomnia remain in a state of hyperarousal, a psychological state marked by anxiety and feeling "on edge." This can further exacerbate blood pressure problems.

Coronary Heart Disease

Prevention of coronary heart disease—the number-one killer of Americans—is a central premise of this book. And sleep can play a role in that. Coronary heart disease is an inflammatory disease, much like lupus. That's because as long as the cholesterol in the plaque remains trapped, there is minimal risk of a heart attack. But if inflammation penetrates the blockage and opens it up, allowing cholesterol to enter the bloodstream, clots can be formed that trigger a heart attack or a stroke.

Research has found that insomnia triggers chronic inflammation, thereby increasing heart-attack risk. In one study, people sleeping fewer than six hours per night had a 20 percent greater chance of a heart attack than people who slept seven to nine hours.

Heart Failure

Heart failure occurs when the heart doesn't pump enough blood to supply the body with the blood and oxygen that it needs to function properly. Studies have found a strong association between insomnia and heart failure. Results from a number of them suggest that people who sleep fewer than seven hours per night have an elevated risk of heart failure. Heart failure was also more common in people who had other indicators of unhealthy sleep in addition to insomnia—including daytime sleepiness, snoring, and being an "evening person." The more of these signs of unhealthy sleep that one person had, the higher their likelihood of heart failure.

Stroke

Ischemic strokes occur when a blood clot or plaque blocks an artery. The same condition in the coronary arteries results in a heart attack.

Research has connected insomnia to a greater likelihood of having a stroke. Insomnia increases blood pressure, and high blood pressure is considered to be the leading risk factor for strokes.

Obesity

People who sleep fewer than seven hours per night are more likely to have a higher body mass index (BMI) or be obese. While more research in this area still needs to be done, some experts believe that insomnia can trigger overeating by influencing the hormones that control hunger.

Type 2 Diabetes

People with diabetes are twice as likely to die from heart disease or stroke than people without this condition. Many factors affect blood sugar, such as diet and weight, but studies have found that a lack of sleep worsens glucose metabolism and is linked to prediabetes.

Obstructive Sleep Apnea

Many sleep disorders have detrimental effects on heart health, but none is worse than sleep apnea. Data from the Sleep Heart Health Study, a National Heart Lung and Blood–sponsored project, indicate that sleep apnea increases the risk of coronary heart disease by 30 percent, the risk of stroke by 60 percent, and the risk of heart failure by a staggering 140 percent!

Obstructive sleep apnea, or OSA, is a breathing disorder that disrupts airflow that occurs primarily as the upper airway collapses when the patient is on his or her back. It often leads to snoring and a reduced level of oxygen in the bloodstream. You don't need to be a cardiologist to recognize that lower levels of oxygen in your bloodstream are a problem. In fact, reduced oxygenation is linked to heart disease, obesity, diabetes, stroke, and high blood pressure.

People with OSA have lapses in breathing during sleep when their airway gets blocked. Interrupted breathing from OSA causes fragmented sleep, which is one reason the condition is tied to multiple cardiovascular problems. In addition, disturbed respiration reduces the amount of oxygen in the blood, which may worsen the impacts of OSA on heart health.

What makes OSA even more relevant to this book is that the condition is also associated with cognitive impairment, making OSA a risk factor for both heart *and* brain health.

DR. SABBAGH: OSA, SLEEP, AND BRAIN HEALTH

A 2018 paper in the journal *Frontiers of Psychiatry* reports that in addition to excessive sleepiness, patients with OSA also experience neuropsychological symptoms such as anxiety, attention deficits, cognitive impairment, depressive symptoms, and other psychological disturbances leading to social adjustment difficulties. Patients diagnosed with OSA demonstrate a decline in a wide spectrum of cognitive abilities, including memory, attention, psychomotor speed, and executive, verbal, and visual-spatial skills. As with the adverse effects of inadequate sleep, this is quite a list!

As you've read, OSA is a major risk factor for heart disease. While it is not a risk factor for Alzheimer's disease, it is a known contributor for cognitive impairment. Studies have linked OSA with impairment of attention, memory, and executive functions. Others have shown that it can negatively affect overall psychological functioning as well as quality of life.

But unlike many other forms of cognitive impairment, we *can* treat it. There are two fairly clear ways to combat OSA.

Both work.

Both are difficult.

The first is CPAP—continuous positive airway pressure. A 2019 study of patients with MCI—mild cognitive impairment—found that adherence to CPAP treatment for one year *significantly* improved cognitive function.

The problem is that adherence to CPAP is low. I've seen it with my patients. They complain about it being uncomfortable and cumbersome. They worry about skin irritation. And in many cases, they express these reservations before they even try it! Studies bear this out. "We have data to show that most patients come to treatment with their minds made up," said Terri Weaver, PhD, RN, of the

University of Pennsylvania School of Nursing, in a 2019 interview about CPAPs with *MedPage Today.*

In February 2021, the FDA approved a new device designed to improve tongue muscle function (which, over time, can help prevent the tongue from collapsing backward and obstructing the airway during sleep).

If you don't like the idea of having to wear a CPAP mask, I sympathize. But please keep this in mind: As I've seen with my patients who did persevere, it'll work. So stick with it.

Or consider another strategy: prevent OSA in the first place. How? By maintaining a healthy weight. Most OSA occurs in BMIs greater than 30. For those who are at that level, consider this yet another reason to lose weight. If you are already maintaining a healthy weight, congratulations—you are also keeping OSA at bay.

Regardless of whether you have apnea or not, a healthy brain requires sleep. And the benefits go beyond the risk of you emitting a hippopotamus-like yawn in the middle of a big meeting—or losing focus while trying to read an important email or follow a conversation.

Studies over the past few years have suggested that sleep helps clear out beta-amyloid, the metabolic waste product found in the fluid between brain cells. (Accumulations of beta-amyloid form the plaques that are one of the hallmarks of Alzheimer's.)

In 2019, a study published in *Science* examined the protein called tau, which accumulates in the abnormal tangles that are also found in the brains of people with Alzheimer's disease. In the healthy brain, active neurons naturally release some tau during waking hours, but it normally gets cleared out of the brain during sleep. "Essentially," the National Institute of Aging put it colorfully in a report on that study, "your brain has a system for taking the garbage out while you're off in dreamland."

The findings suggest that regular and substantial sleep may play an important role in helping delay or slow down Alzheimer's disease. So take out the trash! Get proper sleep for all the reasons we've mentioned. We've asked Dr. Stern, who is also a professor in the Zucker School of Medicine at Hofstra/Northwell, to give us some of her best advice on how to get the rest we need. "We know what the outcomes are from not having enough sleep," says Dr. Penny Stern, MD, MPH, a preventive medicine specialist at Northwell Health in New York. "It's very clear that sleep deficits are linked to many, many problems."

Two studies, both done in Europe and both published in April 2021, underscored the importance of sleep for both heart and brain health. The first, from the *European Heart Journal*, found that disrupted sleep may actually increase your odds of dying early from heart disease or any other cause. Women seemed to be harder hit by these effects than men according to the researchers, who analyzed data from sleep monitors of a total of eight thousand participants. According to a WebMD story on the study, Women who experienced more nightly sleep disruptions over longer time periods had nearly double the risk of dying from heart disease and were also more likely to die early from all other causes compared to women who slept more soundly, the study showed. Men with more frequent nighttime sleep disruptions were about 25 percent more likely to die early from heart disease compared to men who got sounder sleep, the investigators found.

The other study, which garnered national media attention, found that those who got six hours or less of sleep in their fifties and sixties were more likely to develop dementia later in life.

While the authors of this study, published in the journal *Nature Communications*, cautioned that the findings could not link insufficient sleep to dementia, it seems to be a strong factor. "Even though we can't say sleep duration has a causal impact on dementia, it would be good to encourage good sleep hygiene," the lead author, French epidemiologist Séverine Sabia, told the *Wall Street Journal*.

Let the encouragement begin.

"SLEEP IS NOT OPTIONAL": HERE'S HOW TO GET MORE OF IT

In addition to the extensive catalog of adverse health effects we ticked off in the beginning of this chapter, Dr. Stern would like to add a few others. "Accidents, relationship problems, car accidents, poor work performance," she says. "It's a big public safety hazard, too." Sleep fatigue, she says, has been associated with at least 100,000 car crashes and 1,500 deaths each year: "This is a real issue and shouldn't be ignored."

She offers these suggestions for getting better sleep for maximum heart-brain health, starting with a suggestion to take it seriously and not think that somehow, because you are feeling no effects from limited sleep, that you're an exception to this basic human need.

"We're not raccoons, we're not cats," she says. "We're meant to sleep at night. We've had tens of thousands of years of genetic hard wiring that have made us what we are—humans are meant to be awake in the daylight and sleep at night."

So why are you—and so many of us—having trouble sleeping? Because we often resist the signals our body is sending and even fight against them. We switch on lights, we turn on TVs, we allow phones by our bedside to ping and chirp all night long. "Most people don't want to go to sleep when they're tired," she says. "People want to stay up and watch movies, talk-shows or a basketball game."

To get the seven to eight hours most adults need, here are some things you can do:

- *Try to set up a consistent schedule.* As often as possible, try going to bed and getting up at consistent times. "This helps brings your body clock in synchronization," says Dr. Stern.

- *Sleep dark, sleep cool.* Daylight is when you're supposed to be awake. Darkness, when you sleep. So close the drapes (or use blackout curtains if you're working nights). Bears, those famously sound sleepers, seem to understand this better than some of us humans. "Bears hibernate in caves, not on the beach," Dr. Stern points out. Caves aren't hot and stuffy either. "There's a reason people report sleeping better in an air-conditioned room," she says. Your optimal room temperature for sleeping should be around sixty-five degrees.

- *Cover your tootsies.* "I do recommend socks," says Dr. Stern. Several small studies have shown that those who do wear socks to bed fall asleep faster. But she adds, "Even if there is no solid scientific proof as to why socks contribute to better sleep, I've heard anecdotally from many people that socks really do make a difference."

- *Turn off the TV and other technology an hour before you go to bed.* "The thinking is that the desktop, cell phones or TV emit light, which is sending your brain a different message than 'sleep,'" says Dr. Stern. (If you need to keep the cell phone in the room, stick it under the bed.)

- *Instead of texting, try reading.* According to Dr. Stern, reading before bed increases the average person's sleep by fourteen minutes. You can start with this book—and while we hope it won't figuratively put you to sleep, we are happy if it literally aids in the process!

- *Try reading when you* can't *sleep.* "Don't just lay there or toss and turn if you can't sleep," Dr. Stern says. "Getting more and more frustrated about lack of sleep is going to keep you from not sleeping." Instead, she recommends that you get up, leave the bedroom, and go read a book in another room "After a while, you should feel drowsy and that's the time to return to your bed," she says.

- *Consider natural fiber bedding materials.* "Everybody perspires in their sleep," Stern says. Natural fibers—linen, cotton, wool—wick away the perspiration. Synthetic materials do not. "It makes sense to me from a practical point of view," she says. "You want to be comfortable in your sleep and you're going to be more comfortable with natural fabrics." Some studies that have looked at the effects of sleeping on synthetic materials have raised other concerns about the chemicals contained in synthetic fabrics. So Dr. Stern recommends, "Do yourself a favor and use natural fiber bedding."

- *And what about warm milk?* "The old wives' tale used to be that you should drink warm milk to get to sleep better," says Dr. Stern. "Turns out, the old wives might have known what they we're talking about!" Warm milk, she explains, does contain tryptophan and melatonin, which can help you fall asleep. There are other foods rich in these compounds: tart cherries, eggs, fatty fish, and rice are among the best foods to help you sleep, according to the Sleep Foundation (https://www .sleepfoundation.org/nutrition/food-and-drink -promote-good-nights-sleep).

- *Exercise.* Here's yet another reason for physical activity—not an hour before your bedtime, but at some point during the day. "You tend not to find as many sleep problems among routine exercisers," says Dr. Stern.

In sum, don't overlook sleep as a fundamental component of optimal heart and brain health. "You need sleep," says Dr. Stern. "Sleep is not optional, it's essential." Dr. Stern says she often comes across people who seem to think of sleep as a waste of time, an annoyance. "That's a curious way of looking at it," she says. "We all know people who claim that they sleep four or five hours at night, and they're fine. It's really not true. People who routinely achieve good quality and duration of sleep do much better, health-wise."

CHAPTER 8

Step 4

A Sound Approach to Stress Management

I T'S HARD TO OVERSTATE the impact of stress on our lives. Unbridled stress may be the single biggest contributor to illness in the industrialized world. Some experts suggest that 75 percent of diseases and unhealthy conditions are linked to chronic stress. Stress may also be the most misunderstood contributor. It is seldom listed as the official cause of death, but its negative role is undisputed; in fact, experts estimate that mental stress has either caused or aggravated up to 90 percent of all hospital visits in the United States.

As studies show, when you feel like you're in an emotional pressure cooker daily (as half of Americans do), plaque accumulates in the arteries, making blood platelets sticky and prone to forming clots. Arteries begin to constrict, starving the heart of nourishing blood. Meanwhile, as the blood is trying to deal with compromised blood flow, it's also pumping out high levels of cortisol that wear down nervous systems. Chronic stress causes brain shrinkage, particularly in the prefrontal cortex, the area of the brain responsible for memory and learning (more about that later in this chapter).

But you don't have to live life in the stress lane, despite the blinding pace and wrenching changes we have dealt with over the past few years. This chapter reveals some simple adjustments and choices you can make to stress-proof yourself.

First, let's look a little more closely at "stress." And before we look further at its adverse effects—which are legion—let's also not forget that to be stressed is to be human.

"The prevailing idea in our culture is that stress is bad," says University of California, Berkeley (UC Berkeley), biologist Daniela Kaufer. But, she told the *Berkeley Wellness* newsletter, moderate amounts of stress can have benefits: "The stress response is designed to help us react when something potentially threatening happens, to help us deal with it and learn from it."

Those responses, it could be argued, are part of what has enabled our species to evolve. Prehistoric humans may not have needed to get massages or perform deep-breathing exercises to manage stress, but they certainly felt it: the stress of a harsh life, the stress of surviving in a hostile world.

Survive they did, however—and we are the living proof of that. And so while our stress levels today are certainly high, and very different from the eat-or-be-eaten kinds of pressures felt by our distant ancestors, the fact that they overcame these challenges—and that eventually, our species flourished—is proof that we can do that as well.

As society evolved, so did our stresses—and our response to them. Medical observations from the eighteenth century describe people "paled with fear, reddened with rage, or weeping with joy or sorrow." Such observations also noted that people under extreme stress could go mad or pine away from maladies without a clear cause. In 1813, James Johnson, a London physician, was the first to note the impact of chronic stress on health span, describing the relationship between "wear and tear" of life and premature old age. Documentation of the impact of stress on cardiac health goes back even further. Dr. William Harvey, the discoverer of blood circulation, wrote in 1628, "Every affection of the mind that is attended with either pain or pleasure, hope or fear, is the cause of an agitation whose influence extends to the heart." Also recognizing the role of stress, Sir William Osler stated, "My life is in the hands of any rascal who chooses to annoy me." Sir William reportedly died after a heated board meeting at St. George's Hospital in London.

Never has this "agitation" been more evident than in a modern American lifestyle characterized by pressures, time demands, and multitasking. The resulting stress pervades all walks of life. It can be seen in the harried mother at home with young children, the assembly line worker who feels like a cog in a machine, the elderly couple dealing with cancer, the twenty schoolgirls trying out for ten cheerleading positions, the corporate CEO trying to manage a business in a constantly shifting market, and the student who "must" get all As. And of course it can be seen in all of us as we've managed to negotiate life in the pandemic.

Virtually everyone today in American society experiences chronic stress. The pressure of schedules ("I'm late . . . again!") or performance ("I should have done it better and faster") is a common experience. More people are aware of stress as a legitimate lifestyle problem. In one national poll, 89 percent of Americans said they had too much stress in their lives.

But stress is not a stand-alone problem. The emotional turmoil it delivers is connected to anxiety and depression, both seemingly independent factors in elevating cardiac risk. "Stress, anxiety and depression can be viewed as one family of related problems," says Dr. Michael Miller, a psychiatrist at Beth Israel Deaconess Medical Center in Boston.

Incessant stress has a particular negative impact on health span, according to a study published in the journal *Molecular Psychiatry*. This study showed that the powerful stress hormone cortisol changes the way nerves fire, sends circuits into a dangerous feedback loop, and damages the brain. When this happens, it leaves us vulnerable to anxiety, depression, and post-traumatic stress disorder, any of which can compromise health span.

While we often talk about what is stressing us, we may not always be aware of how stress manifests itself in us. Consider some of the following dimensions of stress.

ANGER AND HOSTILITY

Researchers have shown that hostile people—those with high levels of cynicism, anger, and aggression—are at a much higher risk of developing heart disease and other chronic illnesses. "There is something about anger that thickens the walls of the heart and coronary arteries," says Dr. Aaron Wolfe Siegman of the University of Maryland.

Feeling angry from time to time is normal. Anger signals your body to prepare for a fight as part of the "fight or flight" syndrome. Things happen in life that make us mad. Some people express anger readily, shouting and gesturing wildly at the slow driver in the fast freeway lane. Others fume silently over imagined slights. When anger is incurred by a specific event (as opposed to things in general) and is appropriate (a modest level for a moderate amount of time), then it usually is not a health risk. But if anger surfaces too frequently and too intensely and lasts too long each time, and if chronic hostility (in other words, being ready for a fight all the time) begins to take on the look of a personality trait, a commensurate rise in health risk is triggered, particularly for blood pressure, depression, heart attack, and stroke. A number of studies are now showing a link to decreased longevity and health span as well.

We mentioned the unfortunate Sir William Osler, who died after a contentious meeting. He was certainly not the first or last person to succumb almost as a direct result of intense, stress-related hostility. A study at Beth Israel Deaconess Medical Center in Boston reported that the risk of a heart attack increased in the two hours following an episode of anger, suggesting that anger was a trigger that doubled and even tripled heart-attack risk. "Every day in thousands of emergency rooms around the country there are people who have just had a heart attack after arguing with their boss, spouse or children," says Dr. Barry A. Franklin of Beaumont Medical Center. A recent study found that an episode of severe anger was associated with a significantly higher risk of heart attack in the following two hours. Getting so angry that your "blood boils," it seems, may (pardon the pun) end up getting you in really hot water in terms of your heart and arteries.

Physiologically, anger causes stress chemicals like cortisol to be released into the bloodstream. That's a normal response. But again, if anger is chronic and the release of stress hormones is continuous, it can penalize your health by injuring coronary artery walls and stimulating arterial inflammation, blood clotting, and high blood pressure—all of which increase heart-attack risk.

DEPRESSION

Depression is an illness that does more than impact the quality of life; it can shorten your health span and, with it, your life as well. Research suggests that people with major depression tend to live shorter lives than others—and die more quickly than expected when they develop illnesses such as cancer, heart disease, stroke, and diabetes. In one study conducted by the Veteran's Administration, researchers found that patients with depression died, on average, five years earlier than patients without that diagnosis. In addition, compared to other veterans, people with depression lost more years of productive life they might otherwise have been expected to live.

While depression has been linked to a number of chronic conditions, doctors have linked heart attacks and depression for some time, usually in that sequence. After all, who wouldn't be depressed after a heart attack? But new research is showing that depression may be more than a consequence of heart disease; it may actually be a *cause* of it. A number of studies reported that depression preceded a heart attack in up to 50 percent of cases. A study of 4,500 elderly people free of heart disease found that the risk of heart disease and death increased by

60 percent for those who became depressed, compared with 40 percent for those who did not get depressed.

High levels of stress *and* deep depression, described as a "perfect psychological storm," are particularly damaging for people with heart disease. A recent study published in *Circulation* indicates that this combination can raise a heart patient's risk of heart attack or death by 48 percent.

Then there are the so-called Type As. For years, it was believed that these folks—typically characterized as ambitious, impatient, and competitive—were thought to be more susceptible to stress and heart disease than their more relaxed, patient, Type B counterparts. In recent years, psychologists have moved away from the Type A and B designation altogether. "These types do not exist as valid personality constructs, at least not within the scientific field of personality psychology," said Dan P. McAdams, a professor of psychology at Northwestern University, in an article on the website Psycom.

Writing about a 2018 study debunking the Type A/B designation, *Inc.* magazine's Jessica Stillman put it more bluntly. "A complete myth," she declared. "Type A personality doesn't exist."

Another long-held notion now being challenged is that these so-called Type A individuals were more likely to have heart attacks. As it turns out, recent research has found, those who are more competitive, driven, and so forth don't have a greater risk. Hostility—which we just highlighted—is a more accurate predictor.

And, we would submit, so is one's adherence to all the other aspects of good health we've discussed. In other words, a self-identified Type A person (meaning someone who is competitive, ambitious, etc.) who exercises regularly, adheres to a healthy diet, gets proper sleep, and so on, is probably better off in terms of health span than a so-called Type B personality who does none of that!

ANXIETY

Stress, anxiety, and depression are linked together in a toxic mix that can increase cardiac risk and, in doing so, negatively impact health span. Almost 70 percent of people with anxiety disorders also suffer from depression at some point in their lives, and over half the people with depression have an anxiety disorder. They are bound together by chronic stress.

The relationship between depression and heart disease is well established. But now there is mounting evidence for an independent anxiety–heart disease connection as well. People with anxiety disorder seem to suffer from heart attacks more often than those who are not overly anxious.

This is particularly true of people who already have heart disease. While there is much research on the anxiety–heart disease link yet to come, experts point to three results that have emerged so far.

First, people who are anxious often demonstrate unhealthy habits. They smoke, eat a poor diet, and are sedentary. Next, constant anxiety can change the body's "fight or flight" hormonal and physiological response to stress. This in turn can result in high blood pressure, heart rhythm disturbances, coronary inflammation, damage to artery linings, and heart attack. And finally, in a double hit to cardiac health, anxious people tend to have lower levels of protective omega-3 fatty acids and demonstrate an increased propensity for blood clots, both of which increase the risk of a heart attack.

While there is no "one size fits all" treatment for anxiety (treatment can range from medications and exercise to cognitive behavior therapy), many experts agree that managing chronic stress is an effective methodology. We will offer some suggestions on how to do that later in this chapter.

JOE'S JOURNEY: HURRY UP AND SLOW DOWN!

When I was a young man, I had a case of what you could call "hurry-itis": a great sense of time urgency and a desire to do more in less time. I walked fast, talked fast, ate fast, and even turned hobbies into a competition. (Think Cub Scouts boxcar racers!)

Despite my fast-paced life, however, I never got too angry or excited. I was always in a hurry but stayed on an even keel. Anger, hostility, depression, social isolation, and chronic anxiety: none of these, in all honesty, were emotions I felt.

Until *after* my surgery.

That's when I came down with what is often referred to as the "cardiac blues"—a host of negative emotions that affects many heart patients. And it certainly affected me.

In the weeks following my surgery in 1977, I became much more stressed and found myself frequently getting angry. (The blunt opinion rendered by the physician who told me that I probably wouldn't live until age forty didn't help either.)

For about a month, I moped around the house, depressed, anxious, and unable to focus on anything. I had always been actively engaged with life; now I had become a passive observer—except when it came to my heart. In that regard, I was ever vigilant, always on guard for something terrible to happen. One day, on a short walk down the road to our mailbox, I felt a pain in my side and was gripped by panic. It turned out to be nothing more than a muscle cramp, but I believed death was imminent.

There were other behaviors clearly caused by the stress I had put myself under: I became visibly upset when cut off in traffic by another car. I found myself interrupting others in the middle of a sentence or felt a flash of anger when interrupted myself. I became enraged when someone exceeded the maximum number of items permitted in the supermarket express line.

Afterward, I realized that I had become, in some senses, immobilized by stress and fear. And these angry and hostile behaviors, if left unchecked, would lead me exactly where I didn't want to go: back to the hospital.

What became obvious to me was that I needed to manage my stress and not let it manage me. Two techniques that worked well in my case (more are in the second part of this chapter) included regular exercise and positive self-talk. Whether it came from increased endorphins or just blowing off steam, my daily runs and walks around the lake near our home helped keep my stress in line. Mentally, I worked on developing a sense of perspective by utilizing positive self-talk.

That new attitude was put to the test soon after I began to adopt this new posture. I had a flat tire as I was leaving for a meeting. In the past, this would have been the end of the world. But under my new mode of operation, I tried to keep it in perspective. I told myself, "OK, Joe, this is why you have Triple A." Instead of pacing around the car anxiously, waiting for the repair truck to arrive, I sat in my BMW and listened to music.

Part of my new attitude toward stress was recognizing that it couldn't be entirely eliminated. Somewhere along the journey, I heard these wise words: "Life is a little bit like a violin. If the strings are too loose, you can't make any music. If the strings are too tight, you can't make any music."

Upon further research, I learned that the saying is actually attributed to the Buddha. In the most widely accepted version—according to a story published on the website of the Kripalu Center for Yoga and Health—the Buddha is approached by a musician who plays (depending on the translation) a lute or a sitar and is having problems. The player complains that the strings break when he tunes them too tightly. But when they're too loose, the instrument won't produce a sound. Buddha's advice: Find that happy medium. Or, as he says, "Not too tight and not too loose."

Violin, lute, sitar—whatever. The advice still makes sense to me. There needs to be a reason to get up in the morning. There needs to be some stress—positive stress. But if it overtakes your life—if constant stress is making you anxious, depressed, hostile—it's time to take action.

DR. SABBAGH: STRESS AND BRAIN HEALTH

I agree with Joe: trying to live a life without stress is not only unrealistic; it's probably unhealthy as well—for different reasons. We *need* a certain amount of stress in our lives. Our survival as a species has depended on our alertness, our enterprise, our creativity—all our endeavors that to some degree involve stress.

And while we're discussing its effects, perhaps we should define that term a little more precisely, as it's bandied around constantly. "I'm stressed," "This is stressful," "Are you stressed out?"

Let's consider a few definitions. The American Institute of Stress—the very existence of which suggests the magnitude of the problem it poses—acknowledges that there are many different ideas of what the term really means. Two of the most common definitions of *stress*, according to the Institute, are as follows:

- physical, mental, or emotional strain or tension
- a condition of feeling experienced when a person perceives that demands exceed the personal and social resources the individual is able to mobilize

Both of those definitions imply that stress is inherently negative. But let's consider the meaning posited by the authors of a comprehensive review of the effects of stress published in 2017. Stress, they wrote, is "any intrinsic or extrinsic stimulus that evokes a biological response."

That's a broader and more neutral definition. And it makes sense. Think about these events in your life: your wedding day, your graduation, the birth of a child, a big promotion at work. Did any of these red-letter days quicken your pulse, provoke a smile, produce maybe even a few moments of giddy happiness? Probably. By definition, then, they were "stressful." But who would want to eliminate these moments from our lives?

This is why I'm a believer not in stress *reduction* but in stress *management*. There's a difference. I don't know of anyone who is likely to get up tomorrow with less stress. (And if you think you might, just switch on the news!) While it is correct that the term *Type A* is probably outmoded and a bit oversimplistic, you'll forgive me if I use it to suggest that we Americans are a sort of "Type A nation." We are a people who live—and in some cases thrive—under stress. It's in our nature, and while twenty-first-century technology may have intensified our perceived levels of stress, it's nothing new. Do you think that the Founding Fathers declaring independence from Britain or writing the Constitution didn't feel stressed? Or that the pioneers who endured incredible hardships as they explored and settled the West lived stress-free lives?

Granted, as our society has evolved, the perceived levels of stress have probably spiked—to intolerably high levels, in some cases. I see this in my work, and by any definition, it's not the kind of stress that one would want to endure. Those dealing with Alzheimer's are stressed beyond measure. The caregivers are stressed as they try to manage their loved one's treatment. The patients themselves are stressed over their diminishing cognitive skills and gradual loss of autonomy. To that end, an entire department of specialists—psychologists, social workers, and so on—should be available to help as the spectrum of concerns brought forth by patients and families is broad.

Just as the effects of this kind of stress can affect our hearts in the ways Joe explained earlier, it can wreak havoc on many aspects of our brain health. Learning, decision-making, attention, judgment—all of these cognitive abilities have been shown to suffer under the pressure of constant, unyielding stress.

Elements of Stress

Why are we so stressed out about stress if it's a natural and in some ways positive aspect of our survival instinct? As an article on the Mayo Clinic website explains, when you encounter a perceived threat, your hypothalamus, a tiny region at your brain's base, sets off an alarm system in your body. "Through a combination of nerve and hormonal signals," they write, "this system prompts your adrenal glands, located atop your kidneys, to release a surge of hormones, including adrenaline and cortisol."

Cortisol is the main stress hormone, and it plays a helpful role in this initial stress response. But when the "on" switch of this fight-or-flight system gets stuck—in other words, when you constantly feel under attack, under stress—overexposure to this and other hormones can cause serious problems in the brain.

In a 2017 review of the effects of stress published in the *EXCLI Journal*, the authors cited studies showing that chronic stress can actually alter the shape and size of the brain. The hippocampus—one of the brain's key memory centers—seems to be one part of the brain that is particularly affected: the structural changes to the hippocampus include atrophy and neurogenesis disorders, which is why memory is one of the functions most impacted by stress. But cognition—which includes learning, decision-making, attention, and judgment—is also affected by chronic stress. The changes to the stressed-out brain can also be manifested as behavioral, cognitive, and mood disorders.

These effects are not just evident in the elderly either. A 2018 study in the journal *Neurology* found that even among young-middle-age adults, higher levels of cortisol were associated with lower brain volume, impaired memory, and decreased visual perception (interestingly, the association was stronger in women). The researchers even speculated that high stress levels in midlife might be one of many factors that contribute to dementia.

One of the authors of that study, the esteemed neurologist Dr. Sudha Seshadri, MD, jokingly told *Scientific American* that what she and her colleagues found in their investigation "made me more stressed about not being less stressed." But she added, seriously, "An important message to myself and others is that when challenges come our way, getting frustrated is very counterproductive—not just to achieving our aims but perhaps to our capacity to be productive."

Another study, in the journal *Dementia & Neuropsychologia*, went further in drawing the link between stress and senile dementia, concluding that, while the mechanisms are not fully understood, the literature has "extensively shown" that chronically elevated levels of stress hormones play a role in the development of age-related cognitive disorders such as Alzheimer's. But the authors of that study also emphasized that something can be done to alter that outcome: "Given that psychological stress can be managed to a certain extent, learning how to decrease stress levels using evidence-based stress management strategies may be beneficial."

Let's look at some of those strategies now.

Better Stress Management

As you've read, chronic stress is clearly at the intersection of heart and brain health—often in a negative way. But while it penalizes both cardiac and cognitive well-being, one of its most devastating—and perhaps most underresearched—effects is the way in which stress pressures a person into an unhealthy lifestyle. People tend to make poor lifestyle decisions when they're feeling pressured. When under stress, M&M's are lunch. When under stress, we light up cigarettes or have a second or third drink. When under stress, we feel we don't have time to go to the gym.

Thus three of the best things you can do to combat the effects of stress are the steps we addressed in the previous chapters: exercise, eat right, get proper sleep. These actions are good for your brain, good for your heart, and good for managing your stress!

But here are a few more techniques from coauthor Joe Piscatella and others. As he points out, his ability to learn how to manage stress successfully has been instrumental to better cardiac health. "I would not be 40+ years post-bypass without it," he says.

Work in a Work Break

The key to managing stress successfully lies in learning how to produce a relaxation response to offset the stress response. Anything that you can do to relax your mind and body, to disconnect from the hassles of life regularly, will enhance your chances of managing the chronic stress in your life. Says comedian Lily Tomlin, "For fast-acting relief, try slowing down."

This does not happen naturally in our multitasking society; it takes some planning. Joe did it by setting aside time for himself in the midst of a busy schedule to have a break in his day. "Then I performed an activity that helped me switch off, clearing my mind and relaxing," he says. "I'd go for a walk, listen to music, read a book." Never use lack of time as an excuse to keep you from practicing relaxation techniques. "As one person told me, 'I don't *have* the time for a relaxation break, I *make* the time for it.'" Do it for yourself because no one else will do it for you. A relaxation break doesn't have to last for hours. It can take as little as twenty minutes a day.

Make disengaging from screen time a priority. We cited this as a tip for better sleep in the last chapter—it's also a way to better manage stress. You might not be able to do it during the workday, but there should be a time (and preferably it's in the hour or so before bed), where you can step away from the stress-inducing content on your phone or computer.

Breathe Deep!

Deep breathing is a time-honored calming technique in response to a stressful situation; it can also be practiced regularly as a stress preventive, done once or twice a day to break tension's hold. I use it for both purposes.

Most people breathe regularly by expanding the rib cage. This is called chest breathing and results in short, shallow breaths that become most evident when a person is under stress. Unfortunately, it's constricting and has the effect of heightening stress.

A better form of breathing is deep, or abdominal, breathing, which can create a state of calm. The technique is easy to practice and can be done standing, sitting, or lying down. Find a comfortable position and take deep breaths through your nose with your mouth closed. As you inhale oxygen, push out your stomach. This lowers the diaphragm. Hold the breath for a few seconds, and expel it slowly and easily through your mouth with your lips pursed, as if you were whistling or kissing. Make your exhalation twice as long as your inhalation. Both intake and expulsion should be rhythmical. Deep breathing results in slow, regular breaths and creates a state of calmness. Do it for just three or four minutes and tension will dissolve.

"When I first started, I was unfamiliar with this technique and wasn't sure if I was doing it correctly," says Joe. "I found that a good way to learn was to lie on my back and place a weight on my stomach. Two or three books were usually sufficient. When I'd breathe in and push out my stomach, the books would rise; when I exhaled, their weight pressed in. This exercise gave me a good feel for how deep breathing should be practiced. The key to success is doing it daily, in your living room, in your car or at your office. A few minutes each day is all that it takes to bring on the relaxation response."

Try Meditation

Meditation, also called repetition, is a centuries-old technique that involves the repeating of a single word for a concentrated but brief period of time. It is designed to clear the mind and, in doing so, to produce an immediately calming effect on the nervous system. Studies show that when you are asleep, your oxygen consumption is decreased by 8 percent. With meditation, however, it's down by 12 percent, an indication that your body is even more deeply relaxed.

Start by selecting a quiet environment that is pleasant and comfortable. Loosen your clothing if it's tight or uncomfortable and remove your shoes. Assume a comfortable sitting or reclining position, close your eyes, and prepare to focus on something—an object, a word, or your breathing. Empty your mind of everything else.

Take a deep breath and slowly repeat a single word. In *The Relaxation Response*, Dr. Herbert Benson recommends using words or sounds that end in *m* or *n*, such as *calm* or *ocean*, but any appropriate word will do. Slowly repeat the word in your mind over and over again. Other thoughts will occasionally interfere, but just let them pass through your mind.

After a while, the repetition will have an almost hypnotic effect and create a state of deep rest and relaxation. In a few minutes, you'll feel renewed energy and optimism. Like exercise and deep breathing, meditation is a small-step technique that is most effective when done regularly.

Author Deepak Chopra says, "Meditation is not a way of making your mind quiet. It's a way of entering into the quiet that's already there—buried under the 50,000 thoughts the average person thinks every day."

Create a Realistic Perspective

The Chinese character for crisis means "danger," but it also can be translated as "opportunity." This illustrates a tenet basic to an understanding of stress and stress management: it's not the event that is stressful but the perception of the event that produces stress. What may be "danger" to one person is seen as "opportunity" by another. Situations—events, people, to-do lists, and deadlines—are essentially neutral. Of and by themselves, they do not cause stress. Instead, it's one's viewpoint that can make a situation stressful.

Stress—or lack of stress—is the result of perception. Each of us sees the same event differently, and this difference dictates whether the event is stressful. In other words, one person's stress is another person's pleasure. This is illustrated by a story told about a wealthy, elderly woman who, back in the 1960s, lived in a rooftop suite of an elegant hotel in New York. Around one o'clock in the morning, she was awakened by the sounds of a piano in the adjoining suite. Boiling mad at hearing "noise" at that hour, she projected her stress on the front-desk manager, who apologized and explained that the occupant of the adjoining suite was world-renowned concert pianist Arthur Rubinstein. Mr. Rubinstein was disappointed in his performance that evening at Carnegie Hall, and though the audience loved it, he had returned to his suite to replay the entire three-hour concert. Upon hearing the explanation, the woman promptly forgot her complaint, returned to her suite, pulled a chair next to the wall, and spent the next two hours listening to Mr. Rubinstein play!

Had a change of events reduced her stress? No. What had changed was her perception. She had taken a highly charged, stressful event and turned it into one of deep pleasure. What was "noise" at 1 a.m. became beautiful "music" at 1:05 a.m.

The UC Berkeley biologist Daniela Kaufer makes a similar point: it's not necessarily the stress that makes us sick—it's getting stressed out about the stress! "At the end of the day, it's about the appraisal, and dealing with the situation," she says.

Practice Positive Self-Talk

Keeping a straight perspective on events in your mind is aided by a technique called positive self-talk. Each of us is continually involved in an internal conversation that interprets events and actions. Psychologists call these conversations "self-talk." Most people are generally aware of self-talk, although a great deal of it occurs beyond conscious awareness. It takes place in a somewhat automatic fashion, much like riding a bicycle. If you tune in to self-talk, however, you can become more aware of what you are telling yourself and of how self-talk influences your perspective and your feelings.

Some self-talk is positive, such as planning priorities for the next day. Some is neutral, like wondering how long the sermon in church will last. But unfortunately, much self-talk consists of negative, harmful put-downs. If corrected by a boss or parent, we might say to ourselves, "Can't I do anything right?" or "I'm always fouling things up." These messages create a self-perception that increases stress.

Stress is normally viewed as the result of a disturbing event or situation. As seen in the example of the woman and Arthur Rubinstein, however, situations per se are neutral. What really happens when a disturbing event occurs is that we tell ourselves about it: "This is terrible" . . . "How could they do this to me?" . . . "The workload is killing me!" It is this self-talk that triggers the emotion. The process takes place in a step-by-step sequence of events:

A	B	C
Situation →	Self-talk →	Emotion
(A = Antecedent, or the event)	(B = Belief)	(C = Consequences)

Suppose you're scheduled for an important job interview. You jump in your car, turn the key, and—it won't start. The meeting is scheduled for 10 a.m. and there's no way that you'll make it. This is the situation (A). The belief you have about the meaning of the event, your interpretation, takes the form of self-talk (B). In this instance, the talk is negative: "I'm never going to get this job now. They'll think I'm unreliable or that I don't really care about this job. Why does this kind of stuff always happen to me? I'll never have such a great opportunity again."

The result of this is, of course, mushrooming stress (C).

But let's alter that scenario. What if instead of you beating yourself up, the self-talk was *positive,* or at least a more balanced assessment of the situation? "OK, so the battery of my car is dead. Kicking the tires and hitting the steering wheel is not going to help. I'll call an Uber right now, then call the company and explain what happened and that I might be a few minutes late. I'm sure they'll understand. They've probably had the same thing happen many times. And besides, this company wants to interview me. They need to fill the position, and I think they know I'd be a great addition to their staff. Besides, with a little luck, I'll have that Uber here in five minutes, and I really won't be that late after all."

This kind of self-talk produces a very different, and arguably more realistic, perspective of the event and keeps it from generating stress.

The A-B-C model illustrates how thinking influences feelings and explains why two different people can respond to the same situation with far different emotional reactions. It also suggests that emotions can be changed by altering self-talk. This is known as "cognitive restructuring." It calls for being aware of negative self-talk, challenging those self-defeating comments, and replacing them with positive statements that decrease or prevent a negative emotional event.

Positive self-talk is an advertising message for worthiness and control. Like any successful advertisement, repetition is the key—the more often it's repeated, the easier it's remembered.

Try a MindPause

"We live in a constant state of anticipatory angst," says Dr. Carol Scott, MD, describing her day-to-day life as an emergency medicine physician.

Dr. Scott works in the emergency department of a Baltimore area hospital. A modern ER in a major metropolitan area is a stressful place even in the best of times—and these have not been the best of times. In 2020 and 2021, Carol was one of the frontline workers in the fight against COVID-19.

But Dr. Scott is also a certified health and wellness coach—she works with people trying to make personal and positive changes in their lives. She knows full well the importance of physical activity, a healthy diet, and so forth. Yet all the walking in the world can't alter the stressful reality of her workplace during a pandemic. How does she stay calm and composed, particularly in the middle of a day when all hell is breaking loose?

She has developed a technique called MindPause—a sort of planned "time out" from unrelenting stress. She describes it as a "deliberate, decisive disruption from your environment." She emphasizes that MindPause should not be confused with mindfulness. "In the middle of the ER," she says, "I can't go outside and meditate or sit quietly and gaze at the sky. But I can take a MindPause."

Ever watch a movie or a TV show where the scene freezes and the actor turns to address the audience? It's kind of like that. You press pause on everything around you and go, for even just a couple of minutes, to a place of peace and calm. "It's not me visualizing myself at the beach, as nice as that would be," she says. "It's me detached, being non-judgmental. It's me acknowledging the place that I'm in at that moment, and thinking calmly and clearly about the things I need to do next."

There is a multistep process to Dr. Scott's MindPause technique, but here is a very abbreviated version:

- Pause whatever you are doing. Find a virtual and mental space and go there.
- Be aware of what you are experiencing at this particular moment.
- Now that you are in the present moment, identify your current emotional state. Name it. Pay particular attention to any negative emotions.
- Now upload positive emotions instead: vicariously reexperience a meaningful event, situation, or experience in your life "on demand," as if you're choosing from a list of Netflix shows.
- Allow that memory to amplify an authentic, positive emotion (joy, gratitude, serenity, hope, pride, love).
- Recognize any irrational and problematic thoughts. Shift your perspective from problems to possibilities.

In the end, Dr. Scott's view of stress is consistent with those expressed throughout this chapter—that "stress" in and of itself is not necessarily a negative thing. "While high stress may dampen productivity, too little stress can rob individuals of their motivation and drive," she says. Finding your happy medium—what she calls your Best Stress Zone—takes time and a little practice, but as it's a key axis in the intersection between heart and brain health, it's worth your effort.

Just don't get too stressed about it in the meantime.

CHAPTER 9

Step 5

"Cog-Stim" to Jump-Start Your Brain

O N A SUNNY, EARLY spring afternoon in St. Louis, three faces stare out from the darkness of Zoom.

One of them, Jim—who wears a baseball cap sporting the distinctive, redbird-on-the-bat logo of the hometown Cardinals—gazes off-camera with a puzzled look on his mustachioed face.

Mary, who has been helped into her chair in front of their home computer by her husband, Jack, smiles warmly.

Merlin, his distinguished features scrunched into a thoughtful mien, looks as if he's about to listen to a lecture on matters of great importance.

In a sense, that might be true.

"Hi!" says the meeting's cheerful host, Mayra Massey, a doctoral student at Saint Louis University's (SLU's)

Medical Family Therapy Program. She appears young enough to be the granddaughter of those in attendance. "Is everybody feeling pretty good today?"

A brief silence.

"I think so!" ventures Mary.

"Good," says Mayra. "Have you guys been outside today?"

"Huh?" replies Mary, who, like others here, has difficulty hearing, especially on a video conference. "Outside? Yeah, a little bit."

Jim nods.

"How about you, Merlin?"

"Uh . . . not too bad."

"Good, so I thought since last week we talked about going to the zoo and which animals we all liked, I thought today we'd play a little game about things you would prefer to do. Shall we get started?"

"OK!" says Mary, with a supportive, firm nod.

"But first," Mayra says, "I have a song to kick us off."

Mayra hits play on an appropriate tune for a bright and unseasonably warm day: "Here Comes the Sun."

As the familiar melody washes over the group, Mary's smile grows broader. She begins to sing along quietly, mouthing some of the lyrics, gently rocking back and forth.

In some ways, it's been a long, cold, lonely winter indeed for Mary, Jim, and Merlin. But while this weekly meeting of the Cognitive Stimulation Therapy Group—part of the

University's Aging and Memory Clinic—is not going to turn back the calendars for these individuals, all of whom have moderate to severe levels of Alzheimer's and Lewy body disease, the hopeful lyrics would make one think that, at least for this moment, their minds are as clear as the skies invoked in George Harrison's hopeful and beautiful song.

The group, which includes a fourth member, Dan— who arrives, smiling and apologetic, a few minutes later—ranges in age from sixty-six to eighty-five. They're all people who, even just a few years ago, were engaged in careers and family, in meeting the challenges of daily life. All four still live at home, but with a spousal caregiver (for whom this weekly hour provides a much-needed respite as well).

The group has been meeting for nearly three years. "Even as their dementia has progressed, they've been able to participate," says Marla Berg-Weger, PhD, LCSW, executive director of the University's Gateway Geriatric Education Center.

Why? Because while the literature on its effectiveness may not be nearly as strong as for exercise, healthy diet, stress management, and so forth, the "use-it-or-lose-it" logic of cognitive stimulation—"cog-stim," as it's commonly referred to—is difficult to argue, especially in this case. Group Cognitive Stimulation Therapy (CST), a treatment intervention developed in the United Kingdom, aims to keep dementia patients engaged through a range of enjoyable activities designed to spark thinking, concentration, and memory as well as provide the social benefits of being part of a group.

"That's the stimulation part," says Max Zubatsky, PhD, LMFT, the Medical Family Program director at SLU. "When you're in a group setting, you're not only thinking about your own thoughts but tracking other people's thoughts."

Hence the activity for the group today.

"OK, so let's start our Spring edition of 'Would You Rather?'" says Mayra. "Ready?"

"I hope," says Jim.

"Would you rather fly a kite or take a walk?"

Silence. Then Merlin, who has been sitting impassively, chimes in.

"Walk," he says. "I like walking."

"How about you, Mary? Would you like to walk or fly a kite?"

"Oh, that would be fine," she replies cheerfully. "That's very nice."

"Jim?"

Jim looks up at the screen, startled, as if he's been daydreaming. But one can sense him refocusing as he scrutinizes the cartoon images Mayra has put up on the Zoom screen of children flying kites and walking down a street.

"Oh . . . fly!" says Jim decisively.

Similar questions are posed. Would you rather go fishing or feed the ducks?

Skateboard or ride a bike? Play in the dirt or jump in a puddle?

It doesn't seem to matter that these are questions seemingly more relevant to six-year-olds. In fact, having them make decisions on things adults wouldn't likely be doing is deliberate. "It doesn't matter what they answer," says Zubatsky. "It forces them to go to the next level of thinking. They have to imagine what it would be like to do this or that activity in order to answer."

Something that adults can enjoy as well as kids provokes an even more enthusiastic response.

"Would you rather have ice cream or a popsicle?" asks Mayra.

"Well, *there* you go!" declares Dan—as if he's been waiting years for an opportunity to debate this question.

"Popsicle!" says Merlin.

"Ice cream," says Dan.

"Ice cream," agrees Mary.

"What's everybody's favorite?"

"Vanilla!" says Dan.

"Strawberry?" asks Mayra.

"*Noooo,*" says Dan, like the teacher gently correcting a student on an obvious answer. "Vanilla!"

Another musical break: this one for John Denver's "Take Me Home, Country Roads," and again, Mary beams as she sings along—a bit hesitantly, but usually finding the correct words during the chorus. For a moment, one can imagine her as a teenage girl growing up in St. Louis, singing along to this song on an eight-track cassette, the windows rolled down on a summer's day as she drives along Route 66 in her parent's Chevy, with her friends in the back seat, on the way to Burger Chef or to catch a concert at the Arena.

Is that where this song has transported her? To 1971, when "Country Roads" was at the top of the charts? Perhaps—but she must then snap back to the present as the group moves on.

Using activities, examples, or songs that harken back to childhood is also part of the CST plan. "These things reach back to distant memories, and that of course is what people with dementia retain the longest," says Berg-Weger. "Talking about it in the group helps bring those long-age memories back into the present. Whenever you can pull back from the past and bring it forward, that helps them."

If Mary found herself whisked away to the past during the playing of these evocative songs, she certainly didn't remain there. As soon as "Country Roads" concluded, she was ready to answer the next "Would You Rather?" question.

Of course, no one is suggesting that, as a result of their group activities, Mary, Jim, Merlin, or Dave are going to magically regain the sharp minds they had before their disease took hold. But the evidence, both research-based and anecdotal, suggests that they are deriving important benefits nonetheless.

"We've had two of the spousal caregivers say that without this class, they would have likely had to institutionalize their loved one," says Zubatsky.

What's striking when observing the group is not only the protocol; it's the innate kindness and decency of these four individuals—their commitment to the group; their dutiful attention, to whatever degree that is in their power; their willingness, even eagerness, to participate; and the positive energy exuded, particularly by Mary and Dan. All are impressive, and a reminder that plaques and tangles cannot completely strangle a human spirit.

"They always bring a smile to my face," says Mayra, who has been moderating the group since August 2020. "When they have good days and are engaged or remember me, it's always a highlight. They have a special place in my heart."

As the class winds down, Dan—a genial bear of a man and a former high-school football player—wants to make a point about the sporting event he had just been watching on TV that caused him to join the meeting late. "The Four! The Four!" he says. Finally, Mayra asks, "Do you mean the Final Four? The basketball games?"

Dan laughs, "Right!" He then jokingly taps his knuckles on his head in frustration that he couldn't summon the words. "Come out, come out, wherever you are!"

It's both endearing and heartbreaking. And while the value of CST for these individuals is obvious—they clearly enjoy being together—meeting them on Zoom brings one face-to-face with some sobering realities of dementia.

Saint Louis University's program also presents an abject lesson to the readers of this book—part of the purpose of which is to help you better understand and adopt the practices most likely to forestall, delay, lessen the severity of, or even (with luck) avoid the dementia that these good people, and their spouses and families, are battling.

DR. SABBAGH: THE SCIENCE OF STIM

Many experts list what they call *mental exercise* as one of the pillars of brain health.

We would urge people to study, learn, play—and remind them of the value of artistic pursuits. All good ways to build up what we call "brain reserve"— meaning that people who have stimulated and engaged their brains over time will build more connections in their neurons, thus providing a deeper reservoir that can be drawn on to offset some of the inevitable effects of aging.

Cognitive stimulation—cog-stim, for short—makes sense for prevention, for people who want to delay and postpone dementia, and for *you*—someone seeking an optimal balance between brain and heart health to forestall both cardiovascular and Alzheimer's disease. The evidence for this is robust. We know that cog-stim builds synapses and brain connections, enhancing the brain's plasticity, a concept we explored earlier in this book.

Yet while we can wholeheartedly recommend cog-stim (or mental exercise), what we can't offer is a prescription. What we can't give you—as we could with, say, physical activity—are guidelines on the intensity, frequency, or duration with which these activities should be performed. In chapter 5, we detailed the various physical activity guidelines and exercise prescriptions that have been developed over the years. I'm sorry to say that we have nothing like that to offer you for cog-stim. But that doesn't mean we can't both encourage you to integrate mental exercise into your life—and provide some ideas on how to choose those right for you.

Recently, I was part of a committee of medical professionals charged by the UsAgainstAlzheimer's foundation to develop actionable recommendations for clinicians—including talking points they can use as part of the conversations they need to have with their aging patients about cognitive decline—and to suggest to them ways to maintain or improve brain health. After reviewing the literature for cog-stim and following much discussion of our own, we advised them to query patients about their pursuit of the following activities:

- new skills being learned (e.g., cooking, dancing, language, crafting)
- what or how frequently they read

- whether they watch documentaries or news
- making music or creating art
- playing strategy games such as chess
- practicing mindfulness or being exposed to nature

These are all activities that can stimulate your brain. These are all activities that should be encouraged. Thus we encourage *you* to engage regularly in stimulating activities of these kinds.

But as to what might be the next logical questions— Which one of these various cog-stim activities is most effective? How often, and for how long?—I'm afraid that we can't yet offer clinicians, or you, a precise answer.

For example, when you bring up the concept of cognitive stimulation with a layperson, they'll often respond, "Oh, you mean like doing crossword puzzles?" Over the years, that activity has become synonymous with mental stimulation for older adults. And puzzles are indeed a form of cog-stim. But if you do the *New York Times* crossword puzzle every day of the week (and those who are crossword players know that it's designed to get more challenging as the week goes on), does that mean you're getting greater cognitive benefits than someone who does the syndicated crossword puzzle once a week in my hometown paper, the *Las Vegas Review-Journal*?

Maybe, maybe not. And if asked which of these crossword puzzles one should do, or even which one of these publications one should read regularly to help engage one's brain, my answer would be simple: Yes. Yes to both. Yes to either. Yes to doing crossword puzzles. Yes to reading.

I'm not being coy. I'm simply suggesting that when it comes to cog-stim, doing something is definitely better than doing nothing.

That said, are all forms of brain engagement created equal? Let me give you a personal example: my eighty-eight-year-old father recently learned how to speak Spanish. In doing so, did he spark more brain activity than another senior who prefers playing Sudoku? Maybe. But that doesn't mean we should be recommending that every octogenarian go out and learn Spanish if they want to maintain mental sharpness.

As our committee for UsAgainstAlzheimer's recommended to physicians and other medical professionals, "Consider individual and cultural preferences when suggesting activities and discuss different options with each individual to encourage a variety of activities."

I would offer the same suggestion to you: I'm very proud that my octogenarian dad took on the onerous mental task of learning a new language. But suggesting that in order to get the benefits of cog-stim, you need to take a class in computer coding, learn to speak a new language, or read a textbook in thermonuclear physics—well, that's the equivalent of telling you that the only way you can become physically fit is by running a marathon! And while training to run 26.2 miles may be a great goal and a formidable challenge, we know that it's not the only way to get the benefits of exercise—and, in fact, for many people (particularly older folks with joint issues), it might not be the best way.

Same thing here. So far, the findings of those who've researched this question of a "cog-stim formula" have been inconclusive. After reviewing various clinical experiments on this, the authors of one 2011 paper in the *International Journal of Alzheimer's Studies* opined that "perhaps the future of cognitive stimulation interventions relies on the activities practiced in the everyday life of the elderly."

They might be right—and all those activities we listed for clinicians to discuss with their patients (reading, learning new skills, engaging in artistic pastimes) are activities that can be practiced in everyday life. How systemized you need to be, how rigorous you must apply yourself to whatever that activity is, how long you must engage yourself in that activity at any given time to see results—again, we aren't sure.

I would conclude with these observations: whatever you choose to do to keep your brain engaged, make sure it's something you are interested in doing, something you enjoy doing, or something you think you might enjoy trying. The world is full of ways to stimulate yourself mentally. If you don't like playing crossword puzzles, don't start playing them just for cog-stim purposes. You might get bored or frustrated and then stop—thereby defeating the purpose. Rather, find something that interests you; something you've always wanted to explore. And then go for it, as consistently as you can. Cognitive stimulation should be enjoyable as well as beneficial. A bored brain may be almost as unhealthy as an unchallenged one.

One last—and important—point: as this is a book on the intersection of heart and brain health, it's worth noting that a strong link has been found between cognitive impairment and heart failure. A 2019 study in the *American Journal of Cardiology* reported that the prevalence of cognitive decline among patients with heart failure ranges from 25 to 75 percent. Those patients, the authors noted, "experience early death, loss of functional independence, lower adherence to therapy and decreased quality of life." A grim prognosis—and another argument for cognitive stimulation in heart and brain health.

"Cognitive function isn't routinely monitored in patients with heart failure at present," Columbia University's Marco Di Tullio told *Medscape Medical News*. "This is something we need to pay more attention to."

We certainly are—right here, in the pages of this book.

PRACTICAL TIPS FOR STIMULATING YOUR BRAIN FROM AARP

To help choose the right mental exercises for you, AARP's Global Council on Brain Health offers these practical tips:

- *Find something new.* Novelty is important to challenge the brain. If you've already read nine John Grisham novels, and you'd like to make it an even ten, super. But you might also try reading a biography by Ron Chernow or a work of history by Erik Larson; a novel by Hilary Mantel or Alice Munro; thought-provoking, narrative nonfiction by Ta-Nehisi Coates or Malcolm Gladwell. Different topics, different writers mean new and engaging stimuli.

- *Find a brain-training partner.* Pick a skill or hobby that you want to learn and find a teacher, mentor, friend, or companion to learn it from, or with. We'll talk about the benefits of social interaction for brain health in the next chapter, but in terms of compliance alone, having someone else involved can help inspire us and motivate us to keep at it.

- *Practice purposefully.* Building on the previous tip, you might consider an instructor or coach to help you with whatever activity you choose. Being guided by someone who is proficient in the language you want to learn or the instrument you want to play will not only help you improve; their feedback will help keep you motivated to continue.

- *Get schooled.* In a 2018 analysis of the demographics of college students, the *Chronicle of Higher Education* found that about 1.2 million American college students were age forty and over. That number is likely to grow for a number of reasons—including the need for professionals to stay abreast of the fast-changing technologies in their field. If you're still working, maybe taking a class—a serious class on a topic of relevance to your work—would have a double benefit: it would help you on the job, and it would benefit your brain health. If you're already retired, then of course your local college or adult-ed program is filled with classes on all kinds of interesting topics that might stimulate your brain.

• *Make it a little easier on yourself.* Not with the activity itself—the idea is to challenge yourself, after all—but as far as integrating it into your life. In this book, we're encouraging the adoption of a number of healthy behaviors. We recognize that there are only so many hours in the day, and given that about eight of them should be devoted to sleep, finding a cog-stim activity that you can pursue within your schedule—and around your exercise, stress management, and preparation of healthy foods—will increase the likelihood that you will stick with it.

As for what those activities should be, again, it's probably less important *what* you're doing than the fact that you're doing *something.* As author Han Yu of Kansas State University put it in an article in the *Wall Street Journal* on the value of such activities in warding off Alzheimer's, "Live your life as though someone left the gate open. Isn't that what we are supposed to do anyway? If it ends up helping our brains, that's just the icing on top."

THINKING AND MOVING

While he doesn't claim to have invented the term, personal trainer and brain fitness specialist Jonathan Ross calls his approach to cog-stim *neurobics*.

The word has been used by others to describe brain-teasing games, but Ross applies it in a way that seems more genuine and consistent with its roots—a combination of physical and brain exercise.

In chapter 5, we spotlighted the innovative work done by Wichita State University exercise scientist Michael Rogers, with his neural-pathway-activating exercise class for seniors. We also offered some movements by certified personal trainer Bob Phillips that challenged balance and strength, thus involving the neural pathways. Ross, who has won Personal Trainer of the Year awards from both the American Council on Exercise and the IDEA Health and Fitness Association, comes at it from a slightly different perspective: "Most people think of cog stim and they're thinking about learning a new language, solving crossword puzzles and so forth," Ross says. "That's good, but if you look at our brains, they're designed to solve problems in our environment . . . to help us survive. Which usually had to do with producing a specific movement to deal with a specific threat or need."

While the likelihood of one being attacked by a saber-toothed tiger on a morning walk in the suburbs is pretty slim these days, Ross believes that keeping our brains sharp means providing it with stimulating challenges in a physical environment. "It's problem-solving combined with movement," he says.

Thinking and moving, thinking and moving. That's the mantra for Ross when he presents these exercises to his clients. For example, he'll have them roll dice or flip a coin before a workout. "Heads, it's a set of push-ups, tails it's a set of air squats," he says. "You have to think, and then you have to act."

Another example, and one anyone can do, is what Ross calls "letter runs." "Map out a rectangular space in your room or your backyard," he says. "Then you're going to run the letters of your grandchild's name, or run the name of your favorite movie."

Sound easy? Imagine running the letters "s-t-a-r w-a-r-s": navigating the curves of *s*, going side-to-side to cross the *t*, the up-and-down motion to trace a *w*.

"There's a lot of multidirectional running, which is challenging," Ross says, "and you have to stop and think about what those movements would be before each letter. Again, you're thinking and moving."

And of course nonrunners can jog or walk the letters at a more comfortable speed—and still get that neural-stimulating challenge. Ross says you can even practice neurobics on your morning walk as a way to make this most basic and enjoyable form of exercise a little more challenging. "You're out in nature, walking along, maybe listening to music, that's great," he says. "But what if you got out of your regular cadence? What if every few strides, you step off the curve, and then step back on? What if you try to deliberately step on the cracks between the sidewalks? What if you veer off the path and try to weave a figure eight around trees in the park?"

Even doing this for a few minutes, he says, will transform your already-beneficial walk into a more complex—and interesting—activity that will stimulate your brain. "By integrating these cognitive challenges with physical challenges, you're spiking the BDNF even higher," he says, referring to the "brain fertilizer" produced by exercise (which we also discussed in chapter 5). "And you're activating different brain circuits." It's also making both your cognitive stimulation—and your exercise—a little more fun. For more information on Ross's work visit his website www.Funtensity.com.

The value of what he and others, such as Dr. Rogers and Bob Phillips, have done was underscored recently in research showing the surprising benefits of both physical and mental exercise.

The study, conducted at the University of Texas in Dallas and published in *Frontiers in Human Neuroscience*, found that healthy adults who participated in cognitive training demonstrated positive changes in executive brain function as well as a 7.9 percent increase in cerebral blood flow compared to study counterparts who participated in an aerobic exercise program. However, the aerobic exercise group showed increases in immediate and delayed memory performance that were not seen in the cognitive training group—perhaps, the researchers suggested, because those exercises had higher blood flow specifically in the bilateral hippocampi, an area of the brain associated with memory and, the researchers noted, one that is particularly vulnerable to aging and dementia.

"This study highlights the potential to accelerate brain health by adopting lifestyle habits that exercise the mind and body," said Dr. Mark D'Esposito, professor of neuroscience and psychology at the University of California, Berkeley, and one of the study's coauthors.

That's not only a takeaway from that particular study—it's one of the central lessons of this book. To maintain a sharp mind and a strong heart, you need to follow a sound program—a broad, multifaceted program like the one we have presented in this book and that we conclude in the next chapter, where we look at an often-underestimated factor in personal health. And that would be *other people.*

CHAPTER 10

Step 6

Write Yourself a Social Prescription

IN ADDITION TO THE Rx's they routinely (and now virtually) scribble down for medication or therapy, or even those now given for exercise and nutrition, physicians and other health-care professionals in the near future may be adding a new prescriptive recommendation for patients: a social prescription.

Evidence of the power of socialization in forestalling, treating, and managing a wide variety of ailments has mounted over the past few years. This is not just a case of well-intentioned white coats encouraging their patients to get out and see friends a little bit more (which hopefully many will be doing after the pandemic). Social, as opposed to socialized, medicine is more systematic and involves the use of structured group interactions as part of treatment.

"I think it is the way of the future," says UCLA neurologist Dr. Indu Subramanian, a prominent researcher in Parkinson's disease and socialization. "Social prescribing meets people in the community where they are, and links them to social support structures."

This approach is already in evidence in the United Kingdom, where that nation's National Health Service refers patients to so-called link workers, trained specialists who focus on connecting patients to community groups and services for practical and emotional support. Interestingly, link workers not only connect patients with existing groups but also help create new groups, working as needed with local partners.

The power of social support is striking: a 2019 study of Parkinson's patients in five Spanish-speaking countries found that social support was *the* most significant factor influencing quality of life. Another study in 2019 found that having established social support networks was as beneficial to Parkinson's patients as daily physical exercise.

The message is simple: people need to be connected with other people.

As AARP's Global Health Council put it in a special report on "The Brain and Social Connection," "While individuals vary in the degree to which they seek out social connections, humans share a fundamental need to interact with other people. From a brain health perspective, research suggests that older people who are more socially engaged and have larger social networks tend to have a higher level of cognitive function."

Recognizing the importance of this aspect of care, the VA launched in 2020 what they describe as "a new social prescription program" called Compassionate Contact Corp. Originally conceived as a home visitation program for veterans (many of whom had neurological issues), the program was relaunched successfully as a tele-service when the pandemic hit. "Veterans we weren't able to reach with the in-home program, we are able to reach with the 'phone buddy' program," said Prince Taylor, deputy director for VA Voluntary Services. "Sites that were apprehensive about signing up for the in-home program began to sign up for Compassionate Corps." Participation in the program—which involves phone or Zoom calls with trained volunteers—requires a referral from the veteran's medical care team.

Another striking example is one we discussed in a different context in the last chapter: The cognitive stimulation class at Saint Louis University's Memory and Aging Clinic for older adults with mild-moderate dementia. While the benefits of cog-stim are numerous, as we learned, the most important benefit derived from those groups may be, simply, the group interaction. "That socialization part is really key," says Dr. Max Zubatsky, the Clinic's director. "We found that people had improvements using Cognitive Stimulation Therapy—elevated mood, less depression. But those effects were even higher when they were part of a group."

While increasingly seen as a way to manage (or forestall) neurological diseases such as Parkinson's or dementia, the power of socialization, of close relationships and
homogenous communities, also has a storied relationship to heart health—and that story is the one told about
a place called Roseto.

THE ROSETO EFFECT

Located in the Lehigh Valley region of eastern Pennsylvania, Roseto was settled in the late 1800s by immi-
grants from a town of the same name in southern Italy.
In the early 1960s, a time when a great deal of research
and interest was starting to focus on the epidemic of
heart disease in America, Roseto attracted the attention of a team of researchers—led there reportedly by
a chance encounter between Dr. Stewart Wolf, head of
the Department of Medicine at the University of Okla-
homa, and a local physician, who mentioned that the
town had an extremely and unusually low rate of myo-
cardial infarctions—heart attacks. Intrigued, Dr. Stewart
(who had also founded a research lab in nearby Bangor,
Pennsylvania) and a team of researchers investigated the
phenomenon. In a 1964 study published in the *Journal of
the American Medical Association*, they reported some
eye-opening findings about the community of 1,600. It
turned out that for decades, the inhabitants of Roseto had

enjoyed dramatically lower mortality rates from heart disease when compared to other local communities.

How much lower? During the seven years of the study, from 1955 to 1961, for example, there were *no* reported deaths of either sex under the age of forty-seven recorded from heart attacks.

This was astounding. What was the reason?

"It was hypothesized," wrote the authors of a 1992 paper looking back at the original study, "that Roseto's stable structure, its emphasis on family cohesion, and the supportive nature of the community may have been protective against heart attacks and conducive to longevity."

What made the findings even more surprising was that the mid-twentieth-century residents of the town didn't follow what we'd now call "heart-healthy" lifestyles. They ate lots of cheese and sausage (fried in lard, it was reported). They smoked unfiltered cigars. The men worked in foundries, where they inhaled dust and gasses. But apparently all that was offset by something else—a less quantifiable but nonetheless powerful factor that many analysts believe was the real key to the fact that this obscure Pennsylvania community enjoyed such low rates of heart disease.

"No one was alone in Roseto," wrote Dr. Rock Positano in a 2008 article looking back at what became known as the Roseto effect. "Rosetans, regardless of income and education, expressed themselves in a family-centered social life. . . . Families were close knit, self-supportive and independent, but also relied . . . in bad times . . . on the greater community for well-defined assistance and friendly help."

Ironically, by the time the reasons behind the community's seeming imperviousness to hearth disease were being analyzed, things were already beginning to change. "Traditions began to crumble," wrote cardiologist Joel Kahn in a 2020 article. "Children began to move away, attend university, marry outside the community, bring meals in paper bags, and embrace American suburban life. The introduction of a Western lifestyle with long hours of work and social isolation, increased stress, and a processed food diet produced a quick jump in heart attacks and deaths due to atherosclerosis."

Whereas Roseta's residents had enjoyed a rate of heart disease half that of neighboring communities, by the late 1960s, those advantages vanished along with a way of life.

What's the message here? Find a community to live in that still maintains traditional social structures? Live in the same house as your grandparents? Eat more sausage and make sure you fry it in lard first?

No—but it is a reminder of the importance of social connection. The Roseto studies, and the experience of that community, writes Dr. Kahn, suggest that the quality and quantity of our relationships "may be a path to enhance all aspects of the quality of your life." The cautionary tale of the rural Pennsylvania town that defied national trends in heart disease in the 1950s and 1960s—only to reverse direction as its immigrant population became more Americanized—is a lesson for us today. "What Roseto taught us," concluded Dr. Kahn, "is that we humans are social animals who fare best when we're not alone or isolated. The price of modern society in our diet, our stress levels, our exposure to toxins and also our loneliness has been high."

That famous study also reminds us that social connections—whether through family, friends, church, or community organizations or interest groups—may be every bit as powerful as adequate sleep, a good diet, and a regular exercise program for long-term brain and heart health.

JOE'S JOURNEY: BEATING THE "CARDIAC BLUES"

The bluest skies you've ever seen are definitely *not* in Seattle. Although I love living in the Pacific Northwest with the mountains and the water at my back door, the frequent grayness of winter skies can depress me. Going a week or so without sunshine can produce a malaise. Finland has the same problem. I think some of that occurred in the first winter after my surgery.

But while the weather may have been a factor, it was not the main cause of my malaise. As you know from previous chapters, I experienced the "cardiac blues," a postsurgical "down in the dumps" that affects many heart patients. Many experts have linked it to time spent on the heart-lung machine.

I'd describe the "blues" as a combination of sadness over my need for bypass surgery at age thirty-two mixed with anxiety over my future and the potential impact on my family. I also experienced loneliness, as none of my thirtysomething friends could identify with my heart and health situation so I couldn't even discuss my fears and concerns. Thank God for Bernie. Without her constant encouragement, I would have been sunk. She motivated me to learn as much as I could about successfully managing my heart health.

I became immersed in information about heart disease, heart health, cholesterol, medications, diet, exercise, stress, and, yes, the "cardiac blues." Learning about what to do became almost a full-time job for me . . . and it paid off. My biometric measurements—BMI, blood pressure, cholesterol, and such—soon were amazingly good. My cardiologist prescribed me to "keep on doing what you are doing."

While these results gave me a strong sense of satisfaction that eating healthy, exercising regularly, getting enough sleep, and managing stress put me on the right track to heart health, I continued to experience loneliness as a lingering malaise. It became obvious to me then that supporting good heart health was more than just lowering cholesterol and managing blood pressure. An emotional component had to be considered as well.

So I began to research the mind-heart-body connection. The more I researched, the more obvious it was that feelings of loneliness and social isolation, and a lack of social ties, were associated with depression and cognitive decline. That could harm my heart, blood vessels, and brain. I learned about the previously mentioned Roseto effect and other studies as well.

Consider this: one study found that heart-attack survivors scoring high on tests of stress and social isolation were four times more likely to die during the three years after their attacks than those with an expanded social network and little stress. Another found that people with no emotional support who were hospitalized with heart failure had triple the risk of having a heart attack or dying in the next year as those with good support.

On the other hand, studies showed that good social connections can positively influence cardiac health in ways every bit as powerful as adequate sleep, a good diet, and not smoking.

Experts today suggest that while loneliness seems to harm the circulatory system and social connectedness seems to nurture good cardiac health, how that happens is a mystery. It may be that social connectedness somehow influences brain regions that calm the body or put it on high alert.

Once I determined that a lack of social connections could hold me back from optimizing my recovery, the challenge became figuring out what to do.

Over the next few years, I created actions I called "traditions"—things I could do regularly to improve my social connectedness. Here are some of them.

Mended Hearts. This is an organization that has bypass surgery survivors visit patients in the hospital before and after their surgery. It is a support group for patients in need of support, given by those who have "been there." Since there was no Mended Hearts group in my area, I started one. Soon we had over fifty members. This gave me a connection to other bypass patients as we built an organization, developed visiting schedules, and produced a newsletter. It developed a sense of purpose that kept me from dwelling on negative thinking. Their website can be found at https://mendedhearts.org/.

Soccer 1. I had played soccer in school and loved the game, but like many graduates, my postschool exercise consisted of social golf and tennis. That's what I had played prior to my surgery. After the surgery, however, I learned that a men's "over thirty" soccer team was being formed in my town. After getting an OK from my doctor, I rushed to sign up. Soon I was attending practice twice a week and playing games at the local high-school field on Sunday mornings. I loved playing the game, but even more so, I loved being part of a team and having fifteen teammates.

I never spent any time talking to my teammates about my heart condition, but I never felt lonely either.

Soccer 2. My experience with the men's team was so positive that when I was asked to coach a team of five-year-old boys, I agreed. Along with two other coaches who became good friends, I ran practices to teach kids the game and coached them on Saturdays to do their best. Most of all, I had a chance to teach fourteen boys about sportsmanship, team play, and never giving up. I was never lonely while surrounded by these boys, and I coached them for ten years.

Golf. I was never a great golfer, but I enjoyed the social aspect of the sport. So did my best friend, John. So we created a tradition to meet at the golf club at 2 p.m. every Friday. Sometimes we picked up another player, but most of the time it was just John and me playing six, nine, or eighteen holes. The talk, the camaraderie, and the social connectedness never flagged. This was probably the most important and effective tradition that I had.

Coffee. As you've read earlier in the book, since exercise was so important to my heart health, I began to jog (later power-walk) on an everyday basis. This activity, however, could be a lonely discipline. Bernie and I solved this by inviting others to join us for our regular four- to five-mile walk, five days a week, 6 to 7 a.m. After the walk, we went to Starbucks for coffee and conversation. The conversation never flagged as we developed a deep friendship as well as fit hearts.

On Saturdays, we were joined by friends for our walk—sometimes by as many as twenty! Each week, this large group walk would be hosted by a couple who would then supply breakfast to the whole crew. Let me tell you: there's no time to feel malaise, no place for the "cardiac blues," when you're walking along on a bright—OK, even partially cloudy—morning in the Pacific Northwest surrounded by twenty of your friends.

It turns out that my dad had a tradition too, one that began after my mom died and that helped him overcome the social isolation of living the last fifteen years of his life alone. When he passed away at age eighty-six, we were cleaning out his condominium and found 128 sweaters—most of them never worn, many still in boxes from the Nordstrom where he'd purchased them. I remembered at the time that Dad had told me he used to enjoy visiting the Nordstrom at the local shopping mall and chatting with the women who worked there—who obviously didn't mind conversing with a charming old widower. Dad used to tell me about it. "I consider it talk therapy," he joked. And I can tell you that dad did enjoy chitchatting! What I didn't realize is that Dad also felt obliged to make a purchase during his many social interactions with who were then called "sales girls"—most likely to keep them from getting in trouble with any overzealous managers who might have considered their chats with dad to be taking time away from their duties. For dad, I'm sure it was a small price to pay for maintaining an enjoyable source of social interaction.

DR. SABBAGH: SOCIAL STUDIES (AND THE LACK THEREOF)

When I was director of the Banner Sun Health Research Institute, we treated many patients with Alzheimer's and dementia as well as other neurological disorders. It was a busy facility, and no matter what time of day, when I would walk into our facility on West Santa Fe Drive in Sun City, Arizona, the lobby would be packed—but not just with patients or families. Sun City is a major retirement community, and as I learned shortly after starting there, many of those who came to sit in our lobby were there not to be seen or treated by us but just to be in the presence of other humans.

Men, women, some apparently in reasonably good health, others bent and slow-moving with age. They weren't patients of ours (at least not at that point). But they were lonely. They craved any kind of human connection—even just a simple "good morning" or a few pleasantries with strangers. It was heart-wrenching. But it drove home to me the antithesis of what we're talking about in this chapter and what we're recommending to you as part of your heart and brain health.

This was what the lack of socialization looks like. This was loneliness. It's not pretty.

I would not have any hesitation in saying that socialization is an important aspect of health. But as a scientist, I must add that measuring and quantifying its value is difficult. As you have read in previous chapters, we can measure things like memory and cognition and we can measure the effects of exercise and the problems associated with lack of sleep, but I'm not familiar with ways we can clinically capture or quantify social isolation.

While noting the paucity of research, UCLA's Dr. Subramanian—an expert on Parkinson's disease—writes in the journal *npj Parkinson's* that "social isolation is a risk factor for worsened health outcomes and increased mortality. Symptoms such as depression and sleep dysfunction are adversely affected by loneliness."

Things may change in the years ahead as far as our ability to measure and define this aspect of health. Perhaps our colleagues in the social sciences might have tools to help with this and could play a role in the future of developing social prescription protocols in the United States. In the meantime, the authors of a recent *New England Journal of Medicine* article on the U.K. social prescription model agree that better assessment methods are needed. While calling the implications of social prescribing "profound," they noted that "physicians need reliable information on what interventions work best and for whom and how social prescription can best be integrated into conventional medical practice."

That said, I endorse the value of social interaction as one of our pillars of a healthy brain. Even though we can't measure it. Even though I can't pull out a half dozen studies and show you why. Even though I recognize that writing a so-called social prescription (or, technically, an e-prescription in this age of electronic medical records) might be difficult.

Katurah Hartley, a program manager at Cleveland Clinic's Ruvo Center acknowledges that "exactly what a prescription for socialization would look like is a bit nebulous." Still, she, like many others, believes in its value nonetheless. In concert with our center and a statewide initiative called "Dementia Friendly Nevada," Kat and another facilitator hold biweekly "Dementia Conversations" for individuals with mild cognitive impairment. About ten to fifteen people log in on Mondays and Fridays on Zoom to share about the challenge of managing their condition. "We just talk and everyone shares," says Ms. Hartley. "People seem to love it. They're so isolated with their disease, and then the pandemic on top of it, this is a lifeline."

I'm certain that it is. Just as I am certain that staying connected with other people is an essential part of the overall heart and brain health prescriptions we are writing for you in this book. This doesn't mean you have to fill your calendar with activities seven nights a week. That's exhausting! And I fully recognize the value of "alone time." I also realize that some of us are more naturally sociable than others. That's fine—you don't have to be the life of the party (even the Zoom party). You just need to make sure that there is some human connection in your life—preferably based around people and activities you enjoy.

GETTING MORE SOCIAL

"What am I supposed to tell my patients?" one physician said about promoting this aspect of health. "Go out and socialize?"

Well, yes, but admittedly, that may be easier said than done. Especially in the postpandemic world, when more people are likely to spend more time working at home, taking classes at home, and simply being at home. But that's all the more reason to actively look for ways to stay socially connected.

The aforementioned Global Council on Brain Health lists twelve ways you can create more meaningful social engagement in your life:

1. Focus on the relationships or social activities you enjoy the most.
2. If you have no one around who can help you engage socially, turn to professionals who can assist. Examples include telephone hotlines, drop-in centers, a chat with a local religious leader, and so on.

3. If you feel lonely, you can try to change this by making a new connection or by seeking different opportunities to engage with others.

4. If there are barriers to interacting with people (e.g., difficulty getting around, living in an unsafe neighborhood), see if you can identify someone you could ask for help and let someone assist you in making connections.

5. Try to keep a circle of friends, family, or neighbors with whom you can exchange ideas, thoughts, concerns, and practical matters and who can also help or encourage you. It does not need to be a large group of people, as long as those in it are important to you and you are important to them. Try to have at least one trustworthy and reliable confidante to communicate with routinely (e.g., weekly), someone you feel you can trust and you can count on.

6. If you are married, this can benefit your cognitive health, but you should consider fostering other important relationships. Individuals who have never married or are divorced or widowed often have many other connections that provide support.

7. Try to speak every now and then (e.g., monthly) with relatives, friends, and/or neighbors; communicate in person or by phone, email, or other means.

8. Help others, whether informally or through organizations or volunteer opportunities. For example,

visit a lonely neighbor or friend, shop for/with them, or try cooking together.

9. Maintain social connections with people of different ages, including younger people. Keep in touch with grandchildren or volunteer to help people at a local school or community center. Think about the skills you have and that you use routinely that might be valuable to pass on to others. Offer to help teach a younger person a skill you may already have, such as cooking, organizing an event, assembling furniture, saving for the future, investing in the stock market, and so on.

10. Add a new relationship or social activity you didn't try before. Place yourself in everyday contexts where you can meet and interact with others (e.g., stores or parks).

11. Be active and challenge yourself to try out organized clubs, courses, interest groups, political organizations, religious gatherings, or cooking classes.

12. If you are already socially active, diversify your activities. Consider joining or starting a group that doesn't exist in your community and is centered around a common interest (e.g., a workout group).

And finally, here are some additional tips from Joe Piscatella (and although it might have worked for his dad, purchasing excess sweaters is not one of them):

- **Give loneliness a name.** Telling other people you're lonely can feel scary, shameful, and self-defeating.

But expressing that feeling can be the beginning of releasing it.

- **Join a club to make new friends with similar interests.** If you are a heart patient, join a cardiac rehabilitation program. Part of the benefit is sharing information on your recovery actions with other patients.
- **Take time to slow down.** If you're frequently busy, running around with your to-do list, or feel stressed by all the meetings at work, it might be time to hit the brakes. Listen to music, take a bath, or just sit with nothing to do and nowhere to be.
- **Perform anonymous acts of kindness.** Hold a door for somebody or do something nice for a stranger. If you are feeling a bit more extroverted, you might even try starting conversations.
- **Connect daily.** Get out every day and have a conversation, face-to-face, with your neighbor, a friend, your grocer, the librarian—in short, anyone whom you might meet regularly.
- **Volunteer!** Among the many benefits of community engagement is the simple fact that volunteering is a social activity. "Volunteering helps you make new friends!" says the Kiwanis Club. They're right: one of the best ways to meet new people and strengthen existing relationships is to commit to a shared activity. And in the case of volunteering, it's one that will help others as well.

CHAPTER 11

Positive Mental Attitude

The Key to a Strong Heart and a Sharp Mind

THIS BOOK IS DEDICATED to helping people achieve a healthier lifestyle to positively impact cardiac and brain health. That's why a "scorecard" is included: to see where you are now with your health profile and to illustrate that by making the changes we suggest, your current profile can show your progress. The key, of course, is to be able to move from information to action, to turn the advice in this book into real-life habits. In order to do that, you need to develop a positive mental attitude.

There is a two-thousand-year history of the mind-body connection going back to Greek and Roman times. Experts then and experts today counsel that mental outlook can help confer positive physical health and well-being or it can help produce illness. Says Dr. Martin

Seligman, "Positive emotion predicts health and lon-gevity." Much of the choice is up to us. Every day, with-out exception, we find ourselves faced with situations in which we choose how we want to react. We can choose one of two options: a negative reaction (pessimism) or a positive reaction (optimism).

Choosing to react negatively only exacerbates the situation and causes us to lose focus of opportunities to learn and grow. It also can adversely affect our health. Studies show that a negative mental attitude contributes to an increased risk of death from cardiovascular disease, higher rates of depression and anxiety, and increased psychological and physical health problems.

Negativity in attitude can directly impact longevity and health span as well. Studies suggest that negative people have decreased life expectancy. A thirty-year study of 839 patients at the Mayo Clinic, for example, indicated that a pessimistic view was a risk factor for early death, with a 19 percent increase in the risk of mortality.

The opposite is true of a positive mental attitude, which provides benefits to our health and well-being. A study in the American Heart Association journal on six hundred heart patients found that those with positive attitudes exercised more and lived longer. "Thousands of articles in virtually all popular, medical, health and news journals tout the benefits of positive mental attitude on longev-ity, health span and many other positive aspects of aging," says Dr. Peter Norvid, a geriatric specialist at Adventist

Hinsdale Hospital. "Optimistic people live longer, have closer personal relationships and are able to deal with the negative things that happen to them in a way that allows them to continue to be able to be there for others so that others can help them."

A positive mental attitude encompasses the gamut of life's experiences. It's believing in good times during bad times and feeling grateful for what you have instead of lamenting what you lack. It is believing not simply that the positive outweighs the negative in life but that we can create positive feelings and actions—that we have the power to make ourselves happy and content.

As we age, the benefits of having a positive mental attitude are reflected in quantity and quality of life. "When it comes to longevity, a positive attitude is huge," says Ken Budd, former executive editor of *AARP the Magazine*:

> If you believe that life is good, don't you want to experience it? It's clear to me that the people who thrive in their later years are the ones who view each day as an opportunity—to learn, to grow, to savor life. If you're in your late 70s and you're struggling with balance issues that cause you to fall, which approach is better: doing exercises that improve your balance, or confining yourself to a chair? A positive mental attitude fuels us to keep moving, keep doing, keep trying to find the beauty in life. Optimistic individuals are better able to handle the changes that we all face as we age.

Optimistic people are good at putting information into action to create and sustain healthy lifestyle habits.

One thing that becomes obvious in people with an extended health span is that so many of them continue to have a purpose in life, or what one centenarian calls "a reason for getting up in the morning." Having a purpose in life—volunteering, tending a garden, coaching, or taking care of grandchildren—provides a buffer against mortality that supports healthy aging. As one older person said to me, "Age is not a barrier to our dreams and goals. I've met many people who say, 'I'm sixty years old. I can't do this anymore.' I realize that health problems can crop up. But all things being equal, it's attitude that counts. If you're going to think 'I can't do this anymore,' then that's the kind of person you are and will be."

Now, don't get me wrong. Despite what many gurus preach, just thinking positively doesn't cut it. Everyone who accomplishes anything—whether it is writing a book, becoming a top-tier surgeon, or creating an extended health span—accomplishes it the same way: by taking action. Positive people simply have an edge because they believe, they know, that the object of their desire is attainable.

As with many of the other principles we've examined in this book, I learned this one the hard way after my heart attack.

JOE'S JOURNEY: AN ATTITUDE ADJUSTMENT

Despite all the studies and articles linking positive mental attitude to good health, I was not a practitioner of it after my initial bypass surgery. The fact is, I was angry. Here I was, thirty-two years old, raising children, and building a career when, seemingly out of the blue, I became a heart patient needing bypass surgery. What did heart disease have to do with me? It was like having your lotto number drawn only to find that the prize is a firing squad. There was unfairness in life, to be sure. But this felt unfair to the extreme. While our friends were leading "normal" lives, Bernie and I lived for one thing . . . keeping me alive and well.

As you've read, after the surgery, I dedicated much time and effort to understanding how healthy lifestyle habits could help my recovery and to adopting healthy changes in my lifestyle. I did what needed to be done to improve my odds, but I wasn't happy about it. Instead of celebrating a delicious filet of king salmon, I moaned that it wasn't prime rib. Instead of being thankful that I was still capable of running four miles, I was angry that my daily run was virtually mandatory. I didn't really have a choice. For fifteen years, I practiced living healthier as if it were a burden because that's the way it felt.

Let's go back to the time of the surgery, in the summer of 1977. Tests showed that I had a 95 percent blockage of the left main artery—that so-called widow maker. All it would take was a blood clot lodging itself in the small opening and occluding blood flow to the heart, and I'd have a heart attack. The surgeons took a piece of saphenous vein from my leg and used it to create a new arterial channel to my heart. The new channel would allow blood in the coronary artery to flow freely around the blockage. It literally "bypassed" the blocked area, hence the name of the operation.

The use of saphenous veins was "state of the science" in those days. The drawback was that they were veins, not arteries. And that meant that the veins used to create bypasses could not take the wear and tear that arteries can. As a result, the average length of life for a saphenous vein used in bypass surgery was about seven years. If you are eighty or eighty-five years old when you have bypass surgery, seven years may not be such a problem. Not so at age thirty-two.

I was fifteen years post bypass surgery with the original saphenous veins when things turned bad quickly. I've told you about my four- or five-mile morning run (now brisk walk) at the local park. On this morning, I was late for a meeting, so I ran at a fast pace, and as soon as I finished, instead of doing the requisite cooldown—a few minutes to allow your heart to slow down after a bout of vigorous exercise—I finished the run and almost literally jumped into my car and drove off . . . only to completely blackout and awaken with my car on someone's front lawn.

A call was put in to my cardiologist immediately, and I was told to come in right away. Tests showed that my saphenous bypasses were starting to shred. "There is no additional plaque," said the doctor. "In fact, tests show that you have less coronary disease now than fifteen years ago."

I brightened momentarily—this showed that all the changes I'd made were working! But all the king salmon filets and running in the world couldn't change the life-span of that vein, as I realized when he continued: "But this is a structural problem that needs to be dealt with immediately."

So I was wheeled into bypass surgery for a second time, not to bypass a blockage but to replace the saphenous veins with internal mammary arteries. These arteries were now the "state of the science" and could last thirty years or more if good care was taken. While the concept was a simple one that I could understand, the execution brought problems. After the operation, I couldn't seem to come out of a coma-like state. I was awake in my mind but with an unresponsive body. It was a strange feeling: I could hear the bedside conversations but couldn't seem to open my eyes. It was easy to tell from their urgent tones and from the way I felt that things were not going well. I recall the urgent sound of bells and alarms going off frequently: *Were they tolling the minutes to my demise?* I wondered in my dreamlike state.

On the second day of this ordeal, I felt even worse. But even lying in the hospital bed with my eyes closed, my mind was generating negative thoughts: *Why me? Why did this have to happen? I've been working hard to do things right—heck, even the doctor said I'd improved my heart health. And now I'm going to croak despite this? I should have enjoyed that prime rib while I could.*

Still, woozy from the drugs and painkillers, I could hear Bernie conversing with my doctors and my nephew, Todd, and talking on the phone to my son, Joe. Joe and his sister, Anne, were both students at Georgetown University in Washington, DC, some three thousand miles away. Because we didn't want to interrupt their studies and because we expected the surgery to come off without a hitch, they did not come home for the operation.

But things had changed. I was in trouble.

I could also hear Todd—a trusted member of our family—on the telephone talking to Joe Jr. "I don't know how much your mom has told you about the situation here," said Todd, "but you need to come home right now, today."

And after what seemed like a lengthy pause, he added, "And Joe . . . bring a suit."

Bring a suit!

Somehow those words penetrated into my sedated brain. I couldn't believe my ears. I knew what that meant. The battle was being lost. Funeral plans were being made. The businessman in me stirred: *Let's talk about these expenses, and which account they should be drawn from, before anyone gets buried.*

I tried to lift my head and open my eyes, but to no avail. I was alone in my own mind. I realized then that there were two courses of action in front of me. I could take a negative stance—"This is terrible . . . there is no hope . . . I'm fading fast"—or I could project a positive mental attitude centered on the fact that I was still there, with a wife and family that cared and the willpower to turn this situation around.

A picture of me running in the park flashed through my mind, only this time, there was no complaining about the commitment to exercise. I saw it as a positive thing, something I'd like to do for the rest of my life. And so I prayed: "Dear Lord, if I can come out of this with the ability to once more jog in the park, I will never complain about it again."

I'm not saying that God wears Nikes, but I like to think he heard me and decided to give me another chance to rise, to run—to *live*. That was the beginning of the development of a positive mental attitude.

I spent a good portion of the next four days visualizing myself as healthy and whole, and little by little, that visualization became a reality. I opened my eyes and awakened to the smiling faces of Bernie, Anne, Joe, and my nurses and doctors. I knew then that I was going home and Joe could put his suit back in the closet.

Finally, I was ready to leave. I wanted the last night in the hospital, which fell on the anniversary of our engagement, to be a special one for Bernie. I had worked out the logistics with Todd. When Bernie came into my room, I was sitting up in bed with a dress shirt and tie under my hospital gown. On the table were two dinners from our favorite Italian restaurant and a bottle of good wine. Pavarotti sang on the tape deck. It was a special moment and a special night. We were going home!

And thirty years later, my internal mammary arteries are still in place and working—as am I!

FROM KNOWLEDGE TO ACTION

A positive mental attitude is the key to moving knowledge to action. Many people set out with high resolve to make healthy changes after having a health scare, listening to an inspiring speaker, or reading a great article on successful weight loss. "Starting tomorrow," they say, "I'm going to take control of my life, eat better, lose weight, begin an exercise program, and throw away my cigarettes." But most abandon their new program after a few days or weeks. They start strong, but soon their efforts become sporadic and wane, yielding few noticeable results—so they quit. They return to their old, unhealthy habits. Nothing has really changed.

As a motivational speaker, I'm sorry to say that I've seen this happen all too often. Many people institute healthy changes in fits and bursts but fail to turn them into habits and make them a way of life. They have the information needed for the first step—the "why" and the "how" of a healthy lifestyle. But information alone isn't enough to ensure success. According to Thomas Dybdahl, former executive director of the American Prevention Council, people who know that their habits may be unhealthy, and even know what to do, often fail to make changes. "It's hard," he explains. People want instant gratification and fast results. But that's not the way it works with lifestyle changes. "The payoff for losing weight or exercising is way down the road."

The missing ingredient for success is often a positive mental attitude, a basic decision to take action and to persevere until permanent change (a habit) occurs. A positive mental attitude is an outlook that fosters commitment and success, a mental resolve that says, "I'm going to succeed." A good example is a woman I know who lost one hundred pounds—twenty pounds five different times! Each time she would gain the weight back. She had good reasons for losing weight: she wanted to look and feel better and was concerned because her mother, who was obese, was a type 2 diabetic. And after consulting a registered dietician and hiring a personal trainer, she even knew how weight was lost and controlled long-term. What was missing for success was a positive mental attitude, a determination to see change through. "When I viewed losing weight as a problem," she said, "I failed. When I saw it as an opportunity, I succeeded. The difference between failure and success was my attitude."

A positive mental attitude is a perspective that centers on what can be done rather than on what cannot be done. Its importance was illustrated to me in a recent talk I gave to cardiac patients at a large California hospital. After the program, the medical staff introduced me to Vernon and Frank, two patients in their mid-fifties. They were neighbors who worked for the same company and who, ironically, had each undergone bypass surgery in the same month. But that's where the similarity ended. Vernon was doing wonderfully in his recovery. He viewed the changes in his life—healthy eating, regular exercise—as discoveries. He was thankful the surgery had worked so well, providing him with a second chance at an extended health span, and he was determined to live life to the fullest. In fact, he was planning a two-week wilderness hike with his three sons. For Vernon, lifestyle change was a beginning.

Frank, on the other hand, viewed change as an ending. He had become a cardiac casualty. Soon after the operation, he had mentally crawled into a fetal position and thought, *My life is over.* He couldn't do the things he liked to do; he couldn't eat the foods he wanted to eat. In his mind, he was now damaged goods—an old and frail person, fearful of life.

The difference between these men was their mental outlook. For Vernon, change was a stepping-stone; for Frank, it was a roadblock.

I sympathized with Frank. Making healthy lifestyle changes, and turning those changes into longtime habits, is difficult. A positive mental attitude is what helps a person stay committed and persevere one day at a time, keep practicing healthy habits until they become a way of life.

How do we that? Gradually.

SMALL STEPS TO MAKE IT HAPPEN

As with exercise, diet, and stress management, the key to creating and sustaining a positive attitude is by making small steps. Keeping a positive mind-set is difficult if you are trying to do too much too quickly. Failure can drain a positive outlook. For me, successfully establishing a positive mental attitude by using a small-step methodology allowed me to establish and sustain healthy lifestyle habits. Here are some of the small steps I'd recommend.

Set a Time Frame for Good Health

Too often we think of improving health span only as a long-term project, and that can be discouraging and promote a negative attitude. If you need to lose fifty pounds, for example, it seems like it will take forever at the healthy rate of one to two pounds a week. My small-step solution has been to focus on healthy living just for today. If I skipped exercise yesterday or ate a bag of candy, it's over and done. I can't call it back to undo it, so why worry about it? At the same time, I'm not going to be anxious about tomorrow. It isn't even here yet. Instead, I'm going to focus on today, the only day I have and the only day I can control. So I tell myself, "I can't do anything about yesterday and tomorrow, but I know I can make today a healthy one. I know I can schedule a forty-five-minute walk in my day today. I know that I can have a tuna sandwich for lunch today. I know I can be healthy today."

While I am creating a positive mental attitude to make today a healthy one, I try to factor in small improvements in my lifestyle, a kind of "small steps within small steps," to create a heightened sense of success. If my normal exercise is to walk for thirty minutes, I'll go to thirty-five minutes. If I usually drink 1 percent milk, I'll opt for fat-free milk. Making steady improvement feeds my positive mental attitude and builds a foundation for continued success.

The small step of managing my health for today has been fundamental to my healthy aging. Taking one day at a time was reasonable and effective. Pretty soon, the days turned into weeks, then months, and in my case, into forty-forty years. That's a long time to live a healthy lifestyle. But remember, I got there one day at a time.

Get Motivated!

Motivation is fundamental to health-span success because people who don't want to change won't change. It's that simple. Telling them why a healthy change is needed or desirable won't make it take place. All the logical arguments in the world won't make an impact on someone who is not motivated to change. Drs. James Prochaska and Carlo DiClemente in their Stages of Change model describe such a person as in "precontemplation," or not currently considering change (think of "ignorance is bliss"), or in "contemplation," being ambivalent about change (think of "sitting on the fence"). Either way, the person is "not ready" to make changes.

A good example is a man I met about six months after his heart attack and bypass surgery. At the time of the attack, he was seventy-five pounds overweight with a cholesterol count north of 300. Now a half year later, he was in even worse shape. At the request of his justifiably concerned wife, I agreed to talk with him about the importance of healthy lifestyle changes. By the time I arrived for our breakfast meeting at a local restaurant, he had already ordered bacon and eggs, fried hash brown potatoes, toast with butter, and—just to make sure he wouldn't starve until lunch—a side order of pancakes swimming in butter and syrup. It was obvious that he held no interest in eating healthy, and he rationalized his behavior by telling me, "It took sixty-five years for my arteries to get blocked up. If it takes another sixty-five to happen again, who cares?" Down deep, he knew this was not the way that coronary heart disease worked. The simple truth was that he wasn't motivated to make the effort, to do the hard work required, so he made no changes in his lifestyle. In essence, he actively abandoned any effort to secure positive health.

What a contrast to a man I met in a similar situation. A busy executive, he had grappled with chronic stress for many years. His hours were long, so there was never enough time to exercise. He had clients to entertain, which meant a lot of restaurant eating and drinking that resulted in weight gain. He smoked to relax. And he had elevated cholesterol and high blood pressure. The man was a walking time bomb, and one day, the bomb went off. He had a heart attack. I met him about a month after his attack. He was recovering at home and experiencing mental anguish sorting out all the lifestyle changes recommended by the doctors: lose weight; stop smoking; eat a low-fat, low-sodium diet; exercise regularly; practice stress management.

Just thinking about these changes put him on the verge of an anxiety attack. My advice to him was to concentrate less on *what* had to change and more on *why* he wanted to change. My feeling was that if the reasons to change were significant, he would become motivated and find it easier to take the correct action.

I saw him eighteen months later—buying equipment for climbing a mountain with his teenage son! He had lost thirty pounds and was exercising regularly and eating healthfully. He had stopped smoking and was more relaxed. He was spending less time in his office but was so productive that he'd been promoted. He had fundamentally altered his lifestyle.

The reason for his improvement, he told me, was his young family. As he thought of life for them without him, his focus changed. He dwelled less on the unfairness of the situation and became more concerned about what he could do. In a word, he became motivated to change.

One of my books entitled *Positive Mind, Healthy Heart* is a collection of 365 days of quotes, stories, and anecdotes that I've assembled. I still refer to these stories and quotes for my own motivation. This morning, I flipped to one of my favorites, a quote from industrialist Max De Pree: "There are no gold medals for the 95-yard dash."

Outlook Matters

Once in a while, an anecdote says it all. One of my favorites is the one about two salespeople who were sent to the outback of Australia to sell shoes. The salesman emails back to his company, "No potential for sales here. The people don't wear shoes." The second sales rep looks at things differently. His email? "Wonderful potential here. The people don't wear shoes."

The moral of the story: If you view your health as if there are no possibilities for improvement, well, then there are no possibilities. But if you can see those prospects, if you can see hope, if you can see lights at the end of tunnels—you can achieve whatever you envision. Either way, what your mind sees will be right.

Be Open to Change

Change can be hard. Dealing with the unfamiliar and sometimes uncomfortable can arouse fear and breed resistance. Doing things differently takes thought and effort and forces many people out of their comfort zone—the self-image that says, "I am what I am, and I can't change." When faced with a new way of living, reasons not to change are easily found, such as "I know I should eat a high-fiber cereal for breakfast, but my friends meet for coffee and doughnuts every morning and I like being there."

Receptiveness to change is a product of perspective and attitude, an understanding that doing things differently may break a comfortable pattern of life but can result in growth and improvement. A closed attitude, on the other hand, acts as a barrier and prevents the implementation of healthy lifestyle changes. Self-imposed barriers restrict the possible, limit expectations, and impair the ability to change for the better. People have to overcome them in order to see themselves as individuals who *can* live a healthy lifestyle.

I'll use a famous analogy from the sports world: Why did it take until 1954 before the four-minute mile mark was broken? Perhaps it was because no one before Roger Bannister *believed* it could be done. And once he did it, others realized they could do it. Just forty-six days after Bannister broke the four-minute barrier that had stood for decades, an Australian runner did it again. A year later, several milers broke four minutes in the same race. Today, over 1,400 sub four-minute miles recorded, and the world mark is below 3:45. Certainly, technique, training methods, and equipment have improved. But human evolution hasn't changed in sixty-seven years. Once Bannister showed it could be done, everyone knew it was possible for a human to do it again.

This also holds true in making healthy lifestyle changes. If people are locked into the way they've always lived ("I am what I am"), their comfort zone becomes a psychological rut . . . and any attempt to change is met with constant struggle. At best, temporary results are achieved. But if lifestyle change is approached with an open, "can-do" attitude, the chances for long-term success are greatly improved.

Accept Self-Responsibility

Self-responsibility means acknowledging that we alone are responsible for our lifestyle choices and, to a great extent, our heart and brain health. It's easy to blame other people, outside circumstances, or the fact that you are busy as the reasons you're not exercising, not getting enough sleep, not eating right. Other people and our environment do impact our lifestyle, of course, but ultimately, they are not responsible for our decisions and actions. What we do to and for our bodies is a personal responsibility.

This was driven home to me soon after my surgery during a visit with my cardiologist. I had done some research on diet and heart disease, and now, I was ready to take action.

"My diet is a problem, isn't it?" I asked. "Yes, it is," he replied. "Your cholesterol and triglycerides are too high, and you need to lose a few pounds."

"What are we going to do about it?" I inquired. He looked at me and put up his hands. "Darned if I know," he said. "I'm a doctor and I understand disease. If you have another blockage, come back and see me. But you're talking about health, not disease. And frankly, health is not my field."

I was stung by his comments and was so angry that I could hardly speak. But after I thought about it, I realized that he was right. While he could help by providing resources, or directing me to a cardiac rehabilitation program, or recommending a registered dietitian, what he could *not* do was make these positive lifestyle changes for me. He knew I had come to his office looking for a pill or a prescription—a quick fix for my problem. His message, though shocking at first, moved me to a fundamental understanding of who was responsible for the way I lived. It was my heart, my life, my diet—and ultimately, my health. The decisions and actions also had to be mine.

That message was reinforced the following week when I attended a healthy-eating class as part of the hospital's cardiac rehabilitation program. Of the twelve male bypass patients who had been invited, I was the only one who showed up. The other eleven sent their wives! Granted, this was the late 1970s, when gender roles were different. But still, these men did not see themselves as being responsible for what they ate. Instead, they saddled their wives with that responsibility. No one can assume responsibility for another's health. Not only is it unfair; it doesn't work.

Develop Resilience

Everyday life is filled with events that can knock any of us down. We all react to adversity a little bit differently. One person can be devastated by losing a job, while another takes a deep breath and moves on. One person simply collapses under the weight of his troubles, while his neighbor actively looks for a way to get through them and even thrive. That's the resilient and persistent person I want to focus on—the individual who, whatever comes his way, manages to keep control of his thoughts, feelings, focus, and actions. That's the person who, when knocked down, bounces back.

Early on in my small-step journey to a healthy lifestyle, I learned that failure was not found in falling down. True failure is not getting back up again. It's not about missing a workout, staying up late one night to watch a movie and failing to get adequate sleep, or eating a donut. It's about not exercising for a week because you "don't feel like it."

In short, it's about quitting.

Here is a favorite story of mine: A sales manager is firing up his people. "Did the Wright brothers quit?" "No!" they responded. "Did Rocky quit?" "No!" they shouted. "Did Thorndike McKester quit?" There was a long, confused silence. Then a salesperson shouted from the audience, "Who in the world is Thorndike McKester? Nobody's ever heard of him." The sales manager shouted back, "Of course you haven't—that's because he quit!"

Hang in There!

Persevering means stopping not when you are tired but when the task is done. As diplomat and advisor to three U.S. presidents, Robert Strauss once remarked, "It's a little like wrestling a gorilla. You don't quit when you are tired. You quit when the gorilla is tired."

The capacity to persevere is also known as grit, defined as firmness of mind and spirit. It is the ability to dig deep and do whatever it takes to achieve your worthy goals. Sometimes in order to demonstrate true grit, you have to be creative as well as persistent. When Bernie and I were first married, we lived in Tacoma, Washington, but I worked in Chicago. So for a few months, I commuted on weekends until Bernie could join me.

She applied to be a substitute teacher in an elementary school in Chicago and was told by a somewhat curt secretary, "No positions are open. We'll call you if it changes." She went back a half dozen times and always received the same response.

One day, she was home and baked an apple pie. She and I each had a piece at dinner. The following day, having applied yet again and been rejected again, she was so depressed that she ate the whole pie! That did it. It was as if her persistence switch turned on. She marched down to the office and said to the secretary, "You are going to see me here every day of your life. I know you have openings and I'm well qualified to substitute. I'll be here until it happens." An hour later, she was signed up to substitute the following day.

Persistence had gotten her the position, but now she had a pie problem. She did not want her new husband—me—to know that she'd eaten the entire pie. So she baked a new one, ate two pieces, and put the rest on the table for dinner. I gave her props for true grit, but I never learned about her creativity until our twentieth anniversary, when she told me the whole story!

Creating Habits

A positive mental attitude involves a decision to take action and to convert that action into a daily habit. Over time, those daily habits will help you create a healthier lifestyle. Such action first requires the establishment of health goals. Whether you're developing a financial strategy or planning a vacation, to get what you want, you must first *know* what you want. You must have a goal and know where you are headed.

Goals should be specific ("I'm going to lose twenty pounds") rather than general ("I'd like to lose some weight"). This provides direction and a heightened sense of purpose.

It's particularly important to commit goals to writing. Written goals demand clarity, specificity, conditions, a time frame, and a strategy—a process that serves to make the goals "real." It allows a person to prioritize goals so that time and energy can be focused on what is important. Written goals can be measured and reviewed.

Goals also need to be attainable. If you set a goal of losing twenty pounds over, say, ten weeks—a reasonable and healthy rate of two pounds per week—that's realistic. But if someone expects to lose that weight in a month, they're likely to be disappointed.

Goals should reach yet be reachable.

In addition, taking small steps can help turn attitude into action. Instituting a lifestyle for heart and brain health may require changes in a number of key areas. No one should expect to change everything at once. Starting a healthy diet, reducing stress, beginning an exercise program, finding activities to stimulate your brain—to try to accomplish all this at the same time is to invite frustration and failure.

Research suggests that it takes about two to six months to accomplish significant changes and turn them into habits. During that time, a person should not feel pressured to rush or to succeed. Remember, this isn't a race; it's about how you want to live for the rest of your life. The important thing to keep in mind is not the speed of the progress but the continuance of it . . . not quick results but permanent change.

It's been said that health is not something to have but something to become. It recognizes that "becoming" healthy is a process, one in which choices are made and, over time, habits are changed.

Having a positive mental attitude can help inspire you to make the effort to live healthy, to persevere, to succeed.

Remember, the key ingredient is you. Only you can use the information, only you can institute the process, only you can make the choices and changes necessary for good health. Only you can promote your own health. Every time I celebrate our wedding anniversary or pick up a grandchild, I am thankful that I began the healthy lifestyle process over forty years ago. It has provided me with a lifetime of answered prayers.

On behalf of my cowriters, we wish you all the best as you continue to make the changes in your life that will help you achieve the goal of a strong heart and a sharp mind.

Appendix

Menu Ideas for a Heart- and
Brain-Healthy Diet

PREPARED BY TRACY STOPLER, MS, RD,
AND JACQUELINE LEONE

BREAKFAST OPTIONS

Ricotta Toast

- 2 slices whole wheat bread, ½ cup ricotta,
  7 medium strawberries, 1–2 tsp honey, 1 tbsp
  hemp seeds

Avocado Toast

- 2 slices whole wheat bread, ½ avocado mashed,
  ½ cup spinach chopped and mixed into mashed
  avocado, 2 eggs

Yogurt Bowl

- 1 cup low-fat/nonfat/Greek yogurt, ½ cup strawberries, ½ cup blueberries, 1 banana, chopped walnuts or almonds, 1 tbsp hemp seeds

Oats and Yogurt

- ½ cup oats, ⅓ cup yogurt, ½ cup blueberries, 1 banana, ½ strawberries, 2–3 tbsp walnuts

Nutty Oats

- ½ cup oats topped with 1 tbsp nut/seed butter, 1 tbsp hemp seeds, 1 banana

Simple Raspberry Oats

- ½ cup oats, 1 cup milk, ¾ cup raspberries

Tahini Oats

- ½ cup oats topped with 1 chopped banana and 2 dates, 1 tbsp chopped walnuts, 1 tbsp tahini drizzle, and cinnamon

Chia Pudding Bowl

- 3 tbsp chia seeds with 1 cup milk, ⅓ cup (dollop) of yogurt, 1 cup fruit, 1 tbsp chopped almonds

Banana Toast

- 2 slices whole-grain toast, 2 tbsp peanut / almond / sunflower seed butter (any nut/seed butter), 1 sliced banana, 1–2 tsp drizzle of honey, ½ tsp (sprinkle) of cinnamon

Buckwheat Apple Cinnamon Porridge (or Oatmeal)

- ¼ cup buckwheat hot cereal or ½ cup oats cooked with 1 mashed banana, ½–1 tsp cinnamon, ½ chopped apple, topped with 2–3 tbsp chopped walnuts

Egg Scramble

- 2 eggs scrambled with ½ bell pepper, ¼ onion, 2 cups spinach, topped with 1–1½ oz feta or mozzarella

Stuffed Sweet Potatoes

- ½ cup chickpeas roasted in 1–2 tbsp maple syrup and ½–1 tsp cinnamon stuffed into 2 roasted sweet potatoes with 1 chopped banana and 1–2 tbsp almond butter drizzle

LUNCH OPTIONS

Pasta Salad

- 2 oz whole wheat pasta with ½ cup cherry tomatoes, ½ cup red onion, ⅓ cup olives, ½ cup green beans, ½ cup kidney beans, 1 oz mozzarella or feta cheese, 2 tbsp olive oil, juice of 1 lemon, 1 tbsp tahini dressing drizzle

Farro Bean Salad

- ½ cup farro, ½ cup kidney beans, 3–4 cups mixed greens, ½ cup tomato, ½ cup cucumber, ½ avocado, ⅓ cup olives

Chickpea or Shrimp Bowl

- ½ cup quinoa, ½ cup chickpeas, 1 cup mozzarella, ½ cup tomato, ½ cup cucumber, 2 chopped green onions, 1 tbsp parsley, 1–2 tbsp olive oil, juice of 1 lemon, 1 tbsp tahini dressing drizzle

Roasted Chickpea Salad

- ½ cup roasted chickpeas, ½ cup Brussels sprouts, 2 cups chopped kale, ½ cup sweet potato, ½ avocado, 1 tbsp olive oil, juice of ½ lemon dressing drizzle (optional 1 oz feta)

Roasted Chicken Greek Salad

- 4 oz lemon-herb roasted chicken served over Greek salad (3–4 cups mixed greens, ⅓ cup olives, ¼ cup red onion, ½ cup cucumber, ½ cup tomato)

Stuffed Pita Pocket

- Whole wheat pita stuffed with ¼ cup chopped red onion, ½ cup cucumber, ⅓ cup olives, 2 cups spinach, 1–1½ oz feta, ½ cup chickpeas

Spiced Lentil Pita Pocket

- ½ tsp curry spice and ½ tbsp olive oil mixed into ½ cup lentils stuffed in a whole-wheat pita pocket with ½ cup chopped red onion, ½ cup cucumber, ⅓ cup olives, 2 cups spinach, 1–1½ oz feta, 1 tbsp tahini

Caprese Twist Sandwich

- 2 slices whole wheat bread or 1 whole wheat pita, ½ avocado sliced or diced, 1–1½ oz mozzarella cheese, ½ cup sliced tomato, 2 cups spinach, 1 tbsp fresh basil, crack of pepper and salt, topped with 1 tbsp balsamic drizzle

DINNER OPTIONS

Fish with Vegetables

- 3½ oz lemon and herb roasted or grilled salmon/ tilapia/cod/shrimp
  - with 1 cup roasted Brussels sprouts and 1 cup broccoli over 1 cup brown rice/farro/quinoa
  - with 1 cup green beans and 1 cup broccoli over 1 cup brown rice/farro/quinoa
  - with 1 cup roasted Brussels sprouts, 1 cup zucchini, 1½ cups roasted white potatoes, and sweet potato
  - with 1 cup eggplant and 1 cup Brussels sprouts over 1 cup brown rice/farro/quinoa

One-Pan Chicken Roast

- 3½–5 oz chicken breast, 1 cup zucchini, 1 cup eggplant, 1–1½ cup roasted white potato with a lemon wedge to serve

Shrimp Pasta

- 3½–4 oz grilled shrimp with 2 oz pasta, 1 cup eggplant, 1 cup zucchini, 1 cup broccoli in an olive oil lemon sauce (olive oil sauce: 2 tbsp olive oil, juice of 1 lemon, 2 cloves chopped/minced garlic, ½ tbsp dried oregano, and small bunch fresh basil chopped)

Chicken or Shrimp Skewers

- 3½–5 oz chicken or shrimp, ¼ white onion, ½ bell pepper, and 10 baby mushrooms over 1 cup brown rice
- Cut white onion, bell pepper, and mushroom into chunks. Alternate pieces of onion, pepper, mushroom, and chicken pieces on skewers and grill. Once the rice is cooked, chop fresh parsley and mix it into the rice. Serve skewers over the parsley brown rice.

Broccoli Bean Pasta

- 2 oz whole-grain pasta with 1 cup broccoli, 12 cherry tomatoes, 1 cup zucchini, and ½ cup white beans with olive oil sauce (see shrimp pasta recipe)
- Serve pasta and vegetables with a sprinkle of parmesan cheese on top. Sprinkle 1–2 tbsp nutritional yeast over the top for a little extra protein and B_{12} for a nondairy option.

Taco Bowl with Greek Yogurt Sour Cream

- 3½–5 oz ground chicken, ½ cup black beans, ½ cup quinoa, 2 cups romaine, ½ bell pepper, ¼ onion, ¼ cup (dollop) of Greek yogurt to replace sour cream

Fish Mediterranean Tacos

- 3½–5 oz shrimp/salmon/cod, ½ cup cucumber, ½ cup tomato, ¼ cup red onion, ½ cup kidney beans, 3–4 corn tortillas, ¼ cup hummus

SNACK OPTIONS

Roasted Chickpeas

- Makes ½ cup (2 servings)
- 1 can chickpeas
- Lightly coat in olive oil (1–2 tbsp)
- Dust in sweet or savory coating

Sweet Coating

- 1 tbsp maple syrup
- 1 tsp cacao or cinnamon

Savory Coating

- 1 tsp curry seasoning
- Pepper and paprika for a spicy flavor
- Paprika, nutritional yeast, garlic powder, and onion powder for a cheesy chip flavor

Snack Plate

- ½ cucumber, 10–20 baby carrots, 5–10 celery sticks, ½ bell pepper, or any other vegetables of your choosing, ½ cup whole-grain crackers, 1 pita. Serve with your choice of dip.

Nonfat/Low-Fat Yogurt Dip

- Take ½ cup yogurt and add fresh herbs and seasoning (pepper, salt, dill, parsley, cilantro)
- Add 5 tbsp hummus

Yogurt with Fruit and Nuts

- Greek/low-fat/nonfat yogurt with strawberries, blueberries, or banana and walnuts, almonds, or cashews

Apple Nachos

- 1 sliced apple with 1–2 tbsp nut/seed butter drizzle topped with 2 tbsp chopped walnuts and 1–2 chopped dates with a sprinkle of cinnamon

Stuffed Dates

- 2–4 dates stuffed with 2–2½ tbsp nut butter

Chia Pudding

- 3 tbsp chia seeds and 1 cup milk/nondairy milk of choice topped with ¾ cup raspberries and ½ cup blueberries or strawberries

Trail Mix

- 2–3 chopped dates, 2–3 tbsp cashews, 3 walnuts

One-Day Menu for Menstruating Women

Breakfast	Lunch
Avocado Toast 2 slices whole-wheat bread ½ mashed avocado ¼ cup spinach and ½ cup bell pepper chopped and mixed into mashed avocado with the juice of ¼ lime 1 egg on top	**Roasted Chickpea Salad** ½ cup Brussels sprouts 1 cup roasted chickpeas ½ cup sweet potato ½ cup chopped kale 1 oz feta **Dressing** ½ tbsp olive oil Juice of 1 lemon wedge

Dinner	Snack
Salmon Roast 4 oz fish roasted with the juice of 1 lemon, ½ tsp dried oregano, and ½ tsp dried basil with 2 cups roasted broccoli and 1 cup green beans over 1 cup quinoa	**1: Blueberry Walnut Yogurt** ¾ cup Greek yogurt with ½ cup blueberries and 1 tbsp chopped walnuts **2: Carrots with Hummus** 15 baby carrots and 2 tbsp hummus

Nutritional Breakdown

Total Calories	Protein (g)	Protein (%)	Carbs (g)	Carbs (%)	Fat (g)
1807	111.0	23	166.8	48	60.1

Fat (%)	Calcium (mg)	Iron (mg)	Fiber (g)	Sugar (g)	Sugar (%)
29	1096	19.2	56.6	55.7	12

One-Day Menu for Menopausal Women

Breakfast	Lunch
Peanut Butter Banana Oats ½ cup dry oats ½ cup milk ¾ cup water 1 banana 2 tbsp peanut butter 1 tbsp hemp seeds	**Loaded Greek Salad** 1 cup chickpeas ¾ cup farro ⅓ cup chopped tomato 1 cup chopped cucumber ¼ cup chopped red onion ⅓ cup chopped green olives 1 oz feta

Dinner	Snack
Lemon Garlic Salmon 4 oz salmon roasted with 1 clove minced garlic, 1 tbsp lemon juice, salt, pepper 1 cup roasted broccoli 1 cup brown rice	**Cinnamon Raspberry Yogurt** 1 cup Greek yogurt with ½ cup raspberries and ½ tsp cinnamon

Nutritional Breakdown

Total Calories	Protein (g)	Protein (%)	Carbs (g)	Carbs (%)	Fat (g)
1760	106.6	23	178.6	48	58.9

Fat (%)	Calcium (mg)	Iron (mg)	Fiber (g)	Sugar (g)	Sugar (%)
29	923.4	10.9	37.8	50.9	12

One-Day Menu for Men

Breakfast	Lunch
Apple Cinnamon Oats ½ cup dry oats ¼ cup milk 1 cup water 1 medium diced apple 1 tbsp walnuts 1 tsp cinnamon	**Caprese Bowl** 1 cup brown rice ½ cup chickpeas ⅓ cup chopped cucumber ¼ cup chopped olives ¼ avocado 1 oz mozzarella 1 tbsp fresh chopped basil **Dressing** 1 tbsp balsamic dressing ½ tbsp olive oil

Dinner	Snack

Shrimp Tacos
5 oz shrimp
4 corn tortillas
½ cup chopped tomato
¼ cup chopped red onion
½ cup kidney beans
¼ cup corn
1 tbsp fresh chopped parsley
2 tbsp hummus
	1: Tuna Celery Boats
	½ can tuna mixed with ½ tbsp
	   tahini and ½ tbsp mustard
	   stuffed into 8 celery sticks
	
	2: AB&J Yogurt
	1 cup Greek yogurt
	2 tbsp almond butter
	¼ cup strawberries
	1 tbsp hemp seeds

Nutritional Breakdown

Total Calories	Protein (g)	Protein (%)	Carbs (g)	Carb (%)	Fat (g)
2113	133.8	24	205.5	47	71.6

Fat (%)	Calcium (mg)	Iron (mg)	Fiber (g)	Sugar (g)	Sugar (%)
29	1145	14.2	47.4	59.5	11

Acknowledgments

FOR THEIR ENTHUSIASM FOR this project, we would like to thank our literary agent, Linda Konner; Mary E. Glenn, our editor; and the publisher, Humanix Books, as well as Humanix deputy publisher Keith Pfeffer. Thanks also to Lynee Okamoto for helping keep us all connected, Liz Neporent, for her contributions in the early stages of this project and, of course, our family and friends, for all their ongoing support.

A number of medical, health, and fitness researchers and practitioners generously made additional contributions to *Strong Heart, Sharp Mind*. They are identified with their complete titles and affiliations in the book, but we want to briefly recognize them here for providing readers with their perceptive insights and prescriptive advice: Dr. Michael Rogers, PhD; Bob Phillips, CPT; Dr. Penny Stern, MD, MPH; Dr. Carol J. Scott, MD, MS Ed., FACEP; Tracy Stopler, MS, RD, and Jacqueline Leone; Marla Berg-Weger, PhD, LCSW; Max

Zubatsky, PhD, LMFT; Mayra Massey, MMFT; and Jonathan Ross, ACE-CPT.

Finally, as part of the research for this book, we were allowed to pay virtual visits to support group meetings affiliated with Dementia Friendly Nevada and Saint Louis University School of Medicine's Medical Family Therapy Program. Special thanks to Katurah Hartley and her colleagues and participants in Nevada and, in Saint Louis, heartfelt appreciation to Mary and Jack, Jim, Merlin, Dan, and their families and caregivers.

—Joe Piscatella, Marwan Sabbagh, MD,
and John Hanc

Index

About the Authors

JOSEPH C. PISCATELLA is one of the country's most respected experts on how to live a healthy lifestyle in the real world. Through his books, live presentations, and PBS television shows, he has helped improve the lives of millions.

Joe is founder and CEO of the Institute for Fitness and Health, an organization dedicated to helping people initiate and sustain healthy lifestyle habits. *Time* magazine calls him "a positive force for healthy changes." Says Dr. William C. Roberts, editor-in-chief of the *American Journal of Cardiology*, "Joe Piscatella knows more about healthy living and the health impact of our lifestyle choices than anyone I know. He is a national resource."

Joe has written a number of best-selling books, hosted three PBS television specials on heart health, and has been a guest expert on WebMD. As a spokesman for a healthy lifestyle, he has been interviewed on *The Today Show, CNN, Good Morning America*, and *Fox News*.

A professional speaker for thirty years, Joe presents about eighty times a year to medical organizations, corporations, associations, and schools. Over two million people have attended his talks. Joe has served as the only non-medical member of the NIH Cardiac Rehabilitation Expert Panel charged with developing clinical guidelines for physicians. He is also the designer and facilitator of 6 Weeks to a Healthier You®, a successful community wellness program. In one program, 650 people lost a total of 4,200 pounds.

Joe knows the science of healthy living, but he understands the practical aspect as well. At age thirty-two, he underwent coronary bypass surgery. The prognosis was not good (one doctor predicted he would not live to age forty). But he put effort into developing healthy lifestyle habits, and it has worked. He recently celebrated the forty-fourth anniversary of that surgery, making him one of the longest-living survivors of bypass surgery and a shining example of the effectiveness of healthy lifestyle habits.

MARWAN NOEL SABBAGH, MD, board-certified neurologist and geriatric neurologist, hopes to work himself out of a job. Considered one of the leading experts in Alzheimer's and dementia, he has dedicated his career to finding a cure for Alzheimer's and other age-related neurodegenerative diseases.

Dr. Sabbagh is a leading investigator for many prominent national Alzheimer's prevention and treatment trials. He has authored and coauthored hundreds of medical and scientific articles on Alzheimer's research.

Dr. Sabbagh is the author of *The Alzheimer's Answer: Reduce Your Risk and Keep Your Brain Healthy*, with foreword by Justice Sandra Day O'Connor, and of *The Alzheimer's Prevention Cookbook: 100 Recipes to Boost Brain Health*. He edited *Palliative Care for Advanced Alzheimer's and Dementia: Guidelines and Standards for Evidence Based Care* (2010) and *Geriatric Neurology* (2014) and coauthored *Fighting for my Life: How to Thrive in the Shadow of Alzheimer's* (2019).

Dr. Sabbagh earned his undergraduate degree from the University of California, Berkeley, and his medical degree from the University of Arizona in Tucson. He received his residency training in neurology at Baylor College of Medicine, Houston, Texas, and completed his fellowship in geriatric neurology and dementia at the University of California, San Diego, School of Medicine, where he served on the faculty as assistant professor. He has been on the faculty of the Cleveland Clinic, the Barrow Neurological Institute, and the Banner Sun Health Research Institute.

He lives in the Southwest with his wife, Ida Crocker-Sabbagh, MD; his two sons; and their dog, Bowie.

Two of **JOHN HANC**'s most recent books have earned a total of five literary awards. *Your Heart, My Hands: An Immigrant's Remarkable Journey to Becoming One of*

America's Preeminent Cardiac Surgeons (2019), which Hanc wrote with Arun Singh, MD, won four awards, including gold medals in both the 2020 Nautilus Book Awards and the American Society of Journalists and Authors' annual writing competition. *Fighting for My Life: Living in the Shadow of Alzheimer's* (2019), which he wrote with Jamie TenNapel Tyrone and *Strong Heart* coauthor Marwan Sabbagh, MD, also won a Gold Medal in the Nautilus Book Awards.

Hanc writes frequently on health and fitness topics for the *New York Times*, *Newsday*, and *Brain & Life*, the consumer magazine for the American Academy of Neurology. He is a former contributing editor to *Runner's World* magazine, and his articles have also appeared in such publications as *Smithsonian*, *Family Circle*, the *Boston Globe*, and *Columbia Journalism Review*.

Hanc teaches journalism at the New York Institute of Technology and is a member of the faculty at Harvard Medical School's annual Publishing, Editing and Social Media for Healthcare Professionals course.

Simple **Heart Test**

Powered by Newsmaxhealth.com

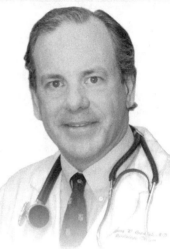

FACT:

▸ Nearly half of those who die from heart attacks each year never showed prior symptoms of heart disease.

▸ If you suffer cardiac arrest outside of a hospital, you have just a 7% chance of survival.

Don't be caught off guard. Know your risk now.

TAKE THE TEST NOW ...

Renowned cardiologist **Dr. Chauncey Crandall** has partnered with **Newsmaxhealth.com** to create a simple, easy-to-complete, online test that will help you understand your heart attack risk factors. Dr. Crandall is the author of the #1 best-seller *The Simple Heart Cure: The 90-Day Program to Stop and Reverse Heart Disease.*

Take Dr. Crandall's Simple Heart Test — it takes just 2 minutes or less to complete — it could save your life!

Discover your risk now.

- **Where you score on our unique heart disease risk scale**
- Which of your lifestyle habits really protect your heart
- **The true role your height and weight play in heart attack risk**
- Little-known conditions that impact heart health
- **Plus much more!**

SimpleHeartTest.com/Strong

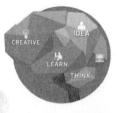

RateMyMemory
Powered by newsmax health

Normal Forgetfulness?
Something More Serious?

You forget things — names of people, where you parked your car, the place you put an important document, and so much more. Some experts tell you to dismiss these episodes.

"Not so fast," say the editors of Newsmax Health, and publishers of *The Mind Health Report.*

The experts at Newsmax Health say that most age-related memory issues are normal but sometimes can be a warning sign of future cognitive decline.

Now Newsmax Health has created the online **RateMyMemory Test** — allowing you to easily assess your memory strength in just a matter of minutes.

It's time to begin your journey of making sure your brain stays healthy and young! **It takes just 2 minutes!**

Test Your Memory Today:
MemoryRate.com/Strong

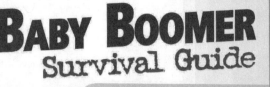